Environmental Safety in the Blood Bank

Editors

Frances L. Gibbs, MT(ASCP)SBB
Supervisor, Immunohematology Reference Laboratory
Associated Regional and University Pathologists
Salt Lake City, Utah

Christina A. Kasprisin, MS, RN
Quality Assurance Coordinator for Nursing
Saint Francis Hospital
Tulsa, Oklahoma

American Association of Blood Banks
Arlington, Virginia
1987

Mention of specific products or equipment by contributors to this American Association of Blood Banks publication does not represent an endorsement of such products by the American Association of Blood Banks, nor does it necessarily indicate a preference for those products over other similar competitive products.

Efforts are made to have publications of the AABB consistent in regard to acceptable practices. However, as new developments in the practice and technology of blood banking occur, AABB's Committee on Standards recommends changes when indicated from available information. It is not possible to revise each publication at the time each change is adopted. Thus, it is essential that the most recent edition of the *Standards for Blood Banks and Transfusion Services* be used as the ultimate reference in regard to current acceptable practices.

American Association of Blood Banks
1117 North 19th Street, Suite 600
Arlington, Virginia 22209

ISBN No. 0-915355-47-7
First Printing
Printed in the United States

Library of Congress Cataloging-in-Publication Data

Environmental safety in the blood bank.

   Based on Environmental Safety in the Blood Bank Technical Workshop, held Nov. 1987 at Orlando, Fla.
   Includes bibliographies and index.
   1. Blood banks—Safety measures—Congresses.
   2. Blood banks—Hygienic aspects—Congresses. I. Gibbs, Frances L. II. Kasprisin, Christina Algiere. III. Environmental Safety in the Blood Bank Technical workshop (1987: Orlando, Fla.) IV. American Association of Blood Banks. [DNLM: 1. Accident Prevention—congresses. 2. Blood Banks—standards—congresses. 3. Occupational Diseases—prevention & control—congresses. WH 460 E61 1987]
   RM172.E58   1987   363.1'94   87-14503
   ISBM 0-915355-47-7

Environmental Safety in the Blood Bank Technical Workshop

Frances L. Gibbs, MT(ASCP)SBB, Director
Christina A. Kasprisin, MS, RN, Codirector

Committee on Technical/ Scientific Workshops

Arthur J. Silvergleid, MD, Chairman

Katherine B. Carlson, MT(ASCP)SBB
Morris R. Dixon, MT(ASCP)SBB
Sandra S. Ellisor, MS, MT(ASCP)SBB
Ronnie J. Garner, MD
Frances L. Gibbs, MT(ASCP)SBB
Sam J. Insalaco, MD
Christina A. Kasprisin, MS, RN
Jerry Kolins, MD
Colin R. Macpherson, MD
Leo J. McCarthy, MD
Jay E. Menitove, MD
JoAnn M. Moulds, MT(ASCP)SBB
Steven R. Pierce, SBB(ASCP)
Alice Reynolds, SBB(ASCP)
Dennis M. Smith, Jr., MD
Stephanie Summers, MEd, MT(ASCP)SBB
W. Michael Tregellas, MT(ASCP)SBB
Virginia Vengelen-Tyler, MBA, MT(ASCP)SBB
Margaret E. Wallace, MHS, MT(ASCP)SBB
Robert G. Westphal, MD

Contents

Foreword

Individuals expect to work in a safe environment. A prudent manager will attempt to create such a work place through appropriate policies and procedures, physical facilities and safety committees. However, a safe work environment cannot be accomplished without the involvement of all employees. In order for the personnel to be active participants in managing the environment, they must be knowledgeable about the risks present and the precautions required in the laboratory setting.

A safe laboratory is the responsibility of all employees. The safety committee is useful in analyzing situations and occurrences that may be indicative of less than optimal conditions.

This text has been designed to provide an overview of safety issues in the blood bank. Chapter 1 discusses the regulatory agencies and laws that govern laboratory safety. Chapter 2 provides a summary of the types of accidents that can occur in the blood bank. Chemicals that are carcinogenic, explosive and ignitable are in use in many laboratories. Chapter 3 describes these chemicals and discusses appropriate precautions. Most workers are aware of the hazards of working with infectious materials. Chapter 4 details the potential viral and other diseases that may be transmitted by blood and discusses methods to safely handle them.

Frances L. Gibbs, MT(ASCP)SBB
Christina A. Kasprisin, MS, RN
Editors

In: Gibbs, FL and Kasprisin, CA, eds.
Environmental Safety in the Blood Bank
Arlington, VA: American Association
of Blood Banks, 1987

1

Compliance with Regulations

E. Shannon Cooper, MD, JD

*T*HE LEVEL OF INTEREST in regulation of laboratory safety is clear, when one considers the number of mandatory and voluntary agencies and organizations involved in this endeavor and the number of employers with programs aimed at improving safety in the laboratory. This chapter will consider how these agencies attempt to regulate laboratory safety in the United States. This examination cannot be comprehensive, and any omission of agencies or other organizations with interests in laboratory accreditation and laboratory safety is unintentional.

Reasons for Regulations

There are many reasons for regulation of laboratory safety in general and blood bank safety in particular. The Senate Committee report prior to the enactment of the Occupational Safety and Health Act described this reasoning eloquently and simply: "Employers have primary control of the work environment and should insure that it is safe and healthful."[1] Clearly, the policy in the United States is that a safe work place for employees must be provided. It is axiomatic that patient and visitor safety is included in this policy. To achieve these ends, regulatory agencies and organizations seek to establish standards of care and practice in many areas of industrial endeavor, laboratories and blood banks included.

If one wonders about the scope of occupational illness as a driving force for regulation of safety, there are multiple sources of information. The starting point would seem to be a definition of what constitutes an occupational disease. Virtually every state has laws containing language defining occupational disease, and

E. Shannon Cooper, MD, JD, Director, Blood Bank, Ochsner Clinic and Alton Ochsner Medical Foundation, New Orleans, Louisiana

many states have been guided by the language that has emanated from court decisions.[2(p 93)] An early court decision (1925) puts forth a definition that is clear and workable:

> *An occupation or industry disease is one which arises from causes incident to the professional labor of the party's occupational calling. It has its origin in the inherent nature or mode of work of the profession or industry, and it is the usual result or concomitant. If, therefore, a disease is not a customary or natural result of the profession or industry, per se, but is the consequence of some extrinsic condition or agent, the disease cannot be impeded to the occupation or industry, and is in no accurate sense an occupation or industry disease.*[3(p 94)]

Although the exact number of occupational diseases and the exact classification of many of these diseases are controversial, there is no doubt that large numbers of workers are exposed to occupational diseases. Doubts can be dissipated by reference to the 67 pages of occupational diseases listed in a book on this subject.[2(pp 293-360)] A somewhat dated report details an astounding number of persons exposed to certain chemicals and other hazards in the United States.[4] Precise numbers are unimportant, but the magnitude of the problem is striking.

As risks are inherent in most occupations, it is unlikely that an employer can ever effect a completely risk-free environment. However, there is a duty, both in common law and created by statutes of the various states and the United States, to eliminate unreasonable risks. Details of some of the statutory regulations of safety will be discussed later. Common law standards and remedies are modified by judicial practice as well as by law-making entities (Congress and state legislatures). Adherence to the standards of care prescribed by statute or by common law is essential for an employer to avoid liability for negligence and even criminal penalties, which may be imposed by statute. Even the animals used in biomedical research have rights protected by Congress.[5]

Sources of Administrative Regulations

To effect the policies of the government of the United States, it was necessary to establish agencies to provide the day-to-day regulation, inspection and other controls needed to accomplish specified ends. Although many organizations provide guidance and require voluntary compliance with standards as an essential requirement for membership and accreditation, federal or state agency control and regulation of laboratory safety are not completely_voluntary. Although the vast majority of businesses and hospitals comply with these regulations on a voluntary basis, they can be enforced through a number of means. The general source of authority for this type of activity comes from the Administrative Procedure Act (APA).[6]

Administrative power is exercised in a variety of ways, the most prominent methods being rule-making and adjudication. Typically, in rule-making, rules become valid only if there is notice and an opportunity for affected parties to comment on the proposal. This type of exercise is sometimes called quasi-legislative, since the "law-making" authority of Congress has been delegated to the agency for specific purposes. The United States Constitution does not establish any agencies, but Congress has done so to effect certain ends of federal law. In addition, some state constitutions also establish agencies. In the federal system, power to administrative agencies is granted by the APA.[6]

Section 553 of the APA details the steps of rule-making, including notice in the *Federal Register* or other personal notice, and the opportunity for affected parties to participate prior to final enactment of the rule. If interested persons wish to participate in the process, they may submit data, opinions or arguments; and, after consideration of these submissions, the agency must incorporate into the rules a general statement of their basis and purpose. This procedure is known as informal rule-making, in contrast to formal rule-making, in which, when it is required by statute, the rules must be based on a record developed during an agency hearing. Formal rule-making is detailed in §556 and §557 of the APA. These procedures comport with general concepts of due process as understood in the United States.

On the other hand, adjudication, when required by statute, must be on record following an opportunity for an agency hearing. The details of the hearing and decision process and exceptions to these requirements are included in §§554-557 of the APA.

Judicial review of agency action is available to any *person* aggrieved or adversely affected by such action.[7] Typically, one must exhaust administrative remedies and the issue must be ripe for review before judicial review is sought. Sanctions for noncompliance are provided for in §558 of the APA; however, sanctions such as the withdrawal, suspension or revocation of licenses cannot be invoked, except in emergencies, without notice and an opportunity for comment.

The Occupational Safety and Health Act

The Occupational Safety and Health Act provides for the establishment of a National Institute for Occupational Safety and Health (NIOSH) and the Occupational Safety and Health Administration (OSHA). The act is found in Title 29 of the United States Code (USC), which is a title related to labor. Accordingly, there is an Assistant Secretary of Labor for Occupational Safety and Health, and the act itself provides authority to administer occupational safety and health standards for all businesses in interstate commerce.

The act provides for five types of standards: Emergency Temporary Standards §655(c), Permanent Standards §655(b), Deemed Standards §655(b)(2), Established Federal Standards §652(10) and National Consensus Standards §652(9). Deemed Standards are those established for specific industries by previous federal legislation and deemed by Congress in the act as an OSHA standard. Established Federal Standards refer to any occupational and safety standard promulgated by any federal agency and in effect when the act was established. The procedures for promulgation of standards and requests for variance from the standards are detailed in the act itself.

The Occupational Safety and Health Act provides specifics for subpoena power, injunctions, citations and other enforcement proceedings.[8] Furthermore, in accordance with the general principles of the APA, there is a provision for judicial review. Of considerable importance to employers (and employees) is §657, which provides for inspections, investigations and record keeping. The authority of OSHA to regulate industrial safety (and by implication, laboratory and blood bank safety) is explicit in this act, and liberal provision of enforcement procedures is provided. Conceptually, employees or employee representatives can request that OSHA inspect and evaluate potential hazards; then, the inspector, as a representative of the agency director, can enforce changes, repairs and the like. Various civil and criminal penalties are detailed in §666, and while not often imposed, they represent a substantial impetus for compliance of a "voluntary" nature.

OSHA has established a Hazard Communication Standard, commonly known as the "right to know" statute, which exemplifies the procedures used by agencies promulgating regulations. In January, 1977, OSHA published in the *Federal Register* (42 FR 5372) an advance notice of proposed rule-making on chemical labeling. Eighty-one comments were received, in general supporting the concept. In January 1981, OSHA published a notice of proposed rule-making entitled "Hazards Identification" (46 FR 4412), but withdrew this in February of 1981 for consideration of alternatives (46 FR 12214). The proposed rule-making was resubmitted in March 1982 (47 FR 12092) and received 221 written comments, which were followed by public hearings in accordance with OSHA's procedural regulations for rule-making (29 FR 1911). Hearings were held in four cities, and a rather large transcript was generated. Post-hearing comments and briefs were also accepted, and the Administrative Law Judge certified the public record in November 1982.

The final OSHA Hazard Communication Standard requires that laboratory employees be apprised of the standards of the chemical products used in their respective work places (48 FR 53331). Although laboratories are exempted from some labeling and other requirements, they are still subject to education and training requirements. Manufacturers, importers and other entities involved with chemical use and handling are also regulated by this final rule. They are required to determine what hazards exist, and they are accountable for the quality of hazard determinations they perform. Potential for adverse effect on health is the primary consideration. The Hazard Communication Standard can be found in the *Code of Federal Regulations* (29 CFR 1910), and interested parties can obtain a copy of the applicable portion of the *Federal Register*, without charge, from the district offices of OSHA. All employers covered by the standard were to have been in compliance by May 25, 1986, although many of the provisions were effective for manufacturers, importers, distributors and some others prior to that date. The *Federal Register* of November 25, 1983, (48 FR 53280-53348) details the final rule. It also provides sources of information used by the agency in promulgating the rule, and suggests sources of information for manufacturers, importers or employers who may wish to obtain additional information about chemicals.

Food and Drug Administration (FDA)

Although the FDA does not purport to regulate laboratory safety directly, the organization has a prominent role in public safety related to food, drugs and cosmetics. The Food, Drug and Cosmetic Act is found at 21 USC §301 et sequitur. The Act provides in some sections (21 USC §§331-337) a definition of crimes associated with violations of the act. In addition, the authority of the FDA to enter and inspect a facility, 21 USC §374(a), is broad. Inspection is limited to reasonable times, and failure to permit an inspection is a prohibited act and a statutory violation (21 USC §331[f]). Penalties can be assessed and warrants as well as judicial orders can be obtained. Seizure of adulterated materials can be accomplished under §334, but parties are entitled to a hearing before the institution of criminal proceedings. The Park Doctrine, enunciated in *United States v Park* 421 US 658 (1975), established a standard for criminal liability of individuals accused of violating the Food, Drug and Cosmetic Act. Basically, the government can proceed when it produces evidence that the defendant had responsibility and authority to prevent or correct violations and did not do so. It is noteworthy that omissions are just as significant as acts in this doctrine.

Department of Transportation

The Department of Transportation regulates the transport of hazardous materials, requiring proper identification, labeling and containers for various hazards. The classification of hazardous material for the purpose of transportation and shipping requirements is found at 49 CFR 172 et sequitur.

Environmental Protection Agency (EPA)

The EPA (42 CFR 261-262) regulates a number of issues related to toxic and hazardous materials. There are civil and criminal penalties for violation of these acts, and to some extent, even the Clean Air Act (42 USC §§7401-7642) is applicable. This requires the EPA to establish national ambient air quality standards for several pollutants. Standards for corrosives and definitions of corrosive materials, ignitable compressed gases, oxidizers, explosives and other hazardous chemicals are found in Title 49 of the *Code of Federal Regulations*.

The US Department of Agriculture (USDA)

The USDA has administrative policies excluding some etiologic agents from the United States. In other cases specific statutes also prevent the importation of particular agents.

Other Forms of Regulation

The Centers for Disease Control, in conjunction with the National Institutes of Health, have recently published a handbook entitled *Biosafety in Microbiological and Biomedical Laboratories.*[9] While the classifications of biomedical laboratories are divided into four levels of biosafety, each with differing criteria and suggested actions, and the handbook does not create a statutory duty to conform to the suggested laboratory practices and techniques, it seems likely that most employers will adopt these measures. Certainly, documents such as this, which are comprehensive and extremely useful, will create a common law standard to which most employers and laboratories would wish to conform. The first edition appeared in March 1984 and can be obtained from the Superintendent of Documents, US Government Printing Office, Washington, DC 20402.

While the Health Care Financing Administration, Medicare and the Clinical Laboratory Improvement Act (42 USC §§262, 263) are concerned more with safety to patients and quality of provision of services, there is an implied standard of safety for employees. Clearly, high quality laboratory work and other services cannot be provided to patients in an environment that is unsafe for employees.

Although many states are involved in laboratory regulation, detailed consideration of state regulations is beyond the scope of this chapter. It is important to note that state regulations cannot preempt federal regulations. It appears that federal regulations can preempt state and local regulations in some areas, but this has not yet been fully applied. *Hillsborough County, Florida v Automated Medical Laboratories, Inc.* (105 S. Ct. 2371) (1985) addressed this point, and this seems to be the law of the land. Conceptually, a local or state government can have regulations more stringent than the federal standard; but, should a federal agency choose to do so, it could probably preempt state and local governments so long as it expresses such an intent. Generally, one must abide by the more stringent of the regulations in order to avoid problems with federal agencies.

Voluntary Regulations

Many agencies are involved in voluntary regulation of laboratory safety. Although this seems somewhat paradoxical, in that regulations are generally not thought to be voluntary, membership and compliance with the standards of these organizations are not required by law but are prima facie evidence of compliance with reasonable standards. Many organizations set standards (regarding electricity, chemicals, compressed gases, etc) that are generally very useful. Typically, these standards are set by knowledgeable people working in the field, which often makes the standards more realistic and practical than other forms of regulation.

As examples in the blood bank area, the American Association of Blood Banks and the College of American Pathologists have long-term interests in laboratory safety. Membership in and inspection and accreditation by these organizations are entirely voluntary, but members must abide by the standards in order to retain their accreditation. In both cases, the standards are supplemented by either Inspection Report Forms or Inspection Checklists that provide detailed information for members as well as inspectors. These organizations function by committees, which can provide guidance quickly in a constantly changing environment and help to achieve the maximum level of employee safety possible.

The National Fire Protection Association has established the Fire Protection Code, National Field Gas Code and the National Electric Code, as well as codes for Ovens and Furnaces, Industrial Furnaces, Industrial Furnaces Special Processing, Blower and Exhaust Systems and many others. The American Chemical Society, the Compressed Gas Association and similar organizations provide handbooks and pamphlets regarding methods of reducing risks associated with specific hazards. Similarly, the National Institutes of Health provide a pamphlet through the Government Printing Office relating to laboratory use of chemical carcinogens.

It is clear from the foregoing that there is an immense effort on the part of government and private voluntary organizations to limit risks to employees, and implicitly to improve safety for patients, visitors and other consumers of services. It is sometimes very difficult to be sure that one is in compliance with all applicable standards and requirements, but it is important that laboratories have a comprehensive safety program as well as dedicated individuals who are willing to spend the appropriate time and effort to identify and control risks to safety. The ultimate payoff comes when an employer has provided employees with the safest work environment possible, a concept fully in accordance with the OSHA mandate. Employees then feel that the employer cares for them and is willing to expend effort to protect them from risks. To do less is risky from a legal and regulatory standpoint, not to mention the moral and ethical considerations. Furthermore, the expense of preventing injury in the work place is usually offset by savings in Workmen's Compensation awards, legal expenses and insurance at a later point.

Employer Responsibility

Therefore, in an attempt to provide a safe work place, employers should ensure adherence to mandatory standards and, to the extent they feel it is appropriate, to voluntary standards. This should help them establish a prima facie case that they are concerned about and involved in prevention of laboratory accidents and have met generally accepted standards. The employees should be warned of risks in accordance with the Hazard Communication Standard and, to the extent an employer believes that it is reasonable, employees should be informed of other hazards. Implementation of comprehensive programs can be difficult and complex at the beginning, because it includes reporting, plans and procedures, inspections and evaluations, controls, ongoing monitoring and sanctions against departments or specific employees who do not adhere to the employer's requirements. Furthermore, an employer must be ready to provide care after accidents or exposures have occurred. It will probably not be possible to make every work place or laboratory completely safe from all risk. However, it is essential that, should they be needed, procedures for handling emergencies and limiting risk of spreading hazards to others, as well as provisions for a comprehensive follow-up plan, be instituted.

Typically, Workmen's Compensation laws limit the liability of the employer to specified amounts for specified injuries and diseases. The policy decision behind this is to encourage quick resolution of work-related injuries, continue the income stream of the injured individual and prevent prolonged litigation with its attendant expenses to the employee who then may not collect his or her rightful damages. To implement this policy, a few states award Workmen's Compensation according to a schedule of diseases, whereas other states rely on state common law as a source of guidance in this area. Workmen's Compensation laws generally exclude ordinary diseases of life, but there are differing views in this regard because ordinary diseases of life are difficult to define and, in many cases, what could be classified as an ordinary disease may be aggravated by working conditions.

Employee Responsibility

The responsible employee should exercise due care and good faith in the reporting and control of accidents. One of the major elements of prevention of work-related injury is conscientious employees and supervisors who identify and report risks. Along the same lines, when an accident occurs, the employee has an obligation to report it, regardless of how minor it may appear, because a similar injury may occur to someone else and be more severe. The importance of careful, involved employees cannot be overestimated.

Summary

In summary, there is extensive laboratory regulation in the United States, although most of it is not directed at laboratories alone. Employers in general are subjected to these regulations, and it is critical that they be followed. Involved employees and employers should also monitor the *Federal Register*, in order to have the opportunity to comment on new proposed rules and regulations. This is part of the American system of government, and those choosing not to participate really ought not to complain too vigorously. The regulations in final form may not reflect an individual's opinion or comments, but the agencies generally do take these into account and, in fact, welcome them.

References

1. Senate Report No. 1282, 91st Congress, 2nd Session, 1970:9.
2. Barth PS, ed. Worker's compensation and work related illnesses and diseases. Boston: MIT Press, 1982.
3. Victory Sparkler and Specialty Co. v Francks, 128 A. 635 (1925).
4. The president's report on occupational safety and health, December, 1973. Washington, DC: US Government Printing Office, 1973:152-61.
5. Animal Welfare Act, 7 USC §2131.
6. 60 Statutes 237-244, 5 USC §§551-559.
7. 5 USC §§701-706.
8. 29 USC §§651-678.
9. Richardson JH, Barkley WE, eds. Biosafety in microbiological and biomedical laboratories. Washington, DC: US Government Printing Office, 1984.

In: Gibbs, FL and Kasprisin, CA, eds.
Environmental Safety in the Blood Bank
Arlington, VA: American Association
of Blood Banks, 1987

2

Prevention of Accidents

Carol Pancoska, PhD, MT(ASCP)SBB

S OME OF THE MOST frequent causes of accidents in the
blood bank include: improperly handled needles and
sharps, broken glass, obstruction of passageways, improperly stored chemicals and combustibles, improper or care-
less use of equipment and lack of preventive equipment maintenance.

Employees may perform their work in an unsafe manner because they lack necessary knowledge or skills, to save time and
effort or to promote physical comfort. Other workers may dis-
regard safety warnings in order to gain group approval.

It is the responsibility of every manager to modify unsafe
behavior, whatever the motivation. This can be accomplished by
1) ensuring that appropriate safety training is given to all employees, 2) conducting refresher courses periodically, 3) being
continuously alert for unsafe acts and potential safety or health
risks and 4) taking prompt corrective action whenever unsafe
acts or hazardous conditions are observed. Furthermore, managers should make available approved safety devices and protective equipment, and train employees in their proper use. In
addition, key aspects of a safety program include instrument
preventive maintenance programs, as well as procedures,
equipment and training to meet emergencies that could reasonably be expected to occur. The prompt assessment, evaluation
and action on all safety suggestions and accidents are essential
for prevention of future accidents.

All blood bank employees are responsible for being aware of
safety hazards, following safety policies and procedures and
reporting all incidents and accidents in order to prevent their
recurrence.

Carol Pancoska, PhD, MT(ASCP)SBB, Administrative Director of
Laboratory Services, Department of Pathology, University of Medicine
and Dentistry of New Jersey, Newark, New Jersey

11

This chapter will review specific types of hazards, control measures, treatment protocols, personal protective equipment and the reporting of safety problems in the blood bank. The role of management in establishing an effective safety program will also be described.

General Safety Rules

The AABB *Technical Manual* states that blood specimens from patients and donors constitute the most serious risk to laboratory workers, and that policies and procedures for protection against hepatitis exposure are sensible precautions. Furthermore, blood bankers are cautioned to avoid unnecessary contact with reagents; especially contact with skin, mucous membranes and open cuts. The procedures and reagents typically used in the blood bank should not pose a health hazard to workers, if a few common sense rules are conscientiously applied[1]:

1. Do not eat, drink or smoke in the laboratory.
2. Do not pipette by mouth.
3. Do not lick labels, chew pencils or put any objects into the mouth.
4. Wear gloves if there are breaks in the skin or if the procedure is likely to result in spillage.
5. Wash hands before leaving the laboratory.
6. Maintain ventilation adequate to avoid inhalation of volatile substances.
7. Clean up spills promptly.
8. Obey regulations designed to protect against fire and explosion hazards.
9. Follow all safety instructions carefully.
10. Perform only authorized procedures. Do not experiment. Personnel in responsible research facilities should review their experimental protocols and inform others in the area of possible hazards.
11. Report all accidents and unusual occurrences immediately.
12. Avoid working alone in the laboratory.
13. Do not allow equipment/procedures to run unattended.
14. Do not allow the storage of food or beverages in any blood bank refrigerator that is used for blood/components, reagents or samples. Do not use laboratory ice for preparing food or chilling drinks. Never use laboratory glassware for eating or drinking.
15. Appropriate warning signs should be posted near any hazardous condition.

16. Store acids and bases separately; store fuels and oxidizers separately.
17. Secure compressed gas cylinders.
18. Require grounded plugs on all electrical equipment.
19. Require that each employee be responsible for keeping his or her work area clean and orderly. Workers using common equipment or areas must share the responsibility for keeping those areas in good order.
20. Do not use blood bank benches, aisles or corridors for storage areas. Clean benches at the end of each shift and whenever spills occur. Keep aisles and corridors clear at all times.
21. Safety equipment such as fire extinguishers and fire blankets are to be maintained, inspected periodically and readily accessible at all times.
22. Discard broken glass into designated, clearly marked containers.
23. Report all accidents and incidents (leaks, spills, equipment malfunctions) to a supervisor.

Safety Hazards in the Blood Bank

If accidents are to be prevented, the hazards that may cause them must be recognized. Safety hazards in the transfusion service or blood processing laboratory are much the same as those found throughout the clinical laboratory, and many apply to the donor room as well. For general laboratory safety guidelines, see the College of American Pathologists' Inspection Checklist[2] and the Joint Commission on Accreditation of Hospitals' *Hospital Accreditation Manual*.[3]

Needles and Sharps

Most accidents caused by needles and lancets used for blood collection occur when employees attempt to recap or destroy needles,[4] or when needles attached to IV sets are left connected to empty blood containers when they are returned to the transfusion service. Needlesticks with contaminated needles provide a mechanism of disease transmission. Clipping needles creates aerosols and contamination of environmental surfaces.[4]

Needles used for blood collection should not be recapped, inserted into bedding or placed anywhere where they could cause an injury. After use, needles should be removed from needle holders and placed directly into rigid plastic containers designed for this purpose. Needles and syringes should be discarded intact into the same type of container. Do not attempt to bend or cut needles.[5]

In order for the containers to be effective in preventing accidents, they must be conveniently placed in areas where blood collection activities are conducted. There should be needle containers inside isolation rooms, on collection team trays, in nursing stations, in the donor room and in outpatient collection stations, so that needles can be discarded safely immediately after use.[6]

Nursing policies and procedures for blood transfusion should specify the proper disposal of needles attached to transfusion sets before blood containers are returned to the transfusion service. Needles attached to donor sets should be disposed of in the same manner as needles used for blood collection or transfusion, in order to prevent injury to employees.

Disposal methods may vary according to local regulations, but should be designed to prevent accidental punctures to employees who handle used needles, to decontaminate them, to prevent aerosolization and to prevent their unauthorized reuse.

First aid procedures to follow in case of accidental needlestick should specify cleansing the wound thoroughly with isopropyl alcohol, covering with a bandage, reporting the accident and following other applicable procedures established by the institution to prevent possible disease transmission.[6]

Electrical Hazards

Electrical hazards in the blood bank may cause electrical shock, fire and the ignition of flammable vapors and gases.

Electrical shock can cause burns, painful muscular contractions, ventricular fibrillation and death. As little as 0.001 ampere of 60-Hz current can cause death if it passes through vital organs. The belief that low voltage (<120 volts) cannot injure a person is misleading. A low voltage shock may cause falls, or contact with moving equipment. Furthermore, the resistance of persons to voltage is highly variable among individuals, and depends on the parts of the body affected. The danger is increased when the skin is wet or broken. Current flow, voltage and contact time are the critical factors. Human responses to alternating current can be roughly classified as follows[7]:
1. Perception current (slight tingling sensation) = 1.1 mA in men, 0.7 mA in women.

2. Let go current (one can release the conductor using muscles directly affected by the current) = 15 mA in men, 10.5 mA in women.
3. Lethal current (chest muscle contraction and inability to breathe) = 18 mA.

Death may result from muscular contraction of heart and/or chest, paralysis of nerve centers, ventricular fibrillation, respiratory inhibition or deep burns.

Electrical hazards in the blood bank may include some of these common causes of electrical accidents: frayed wiring or short circuits, overloaded outlets, improperly grounded equipment, water or saline accumulating on floors or bench tops on which instruments are operating, attempting to repair instruments while they are on and attempting to repair instruments while wearing conductive rings, watches or glasses frames.

Good facility design and maintenance, as well as periodic inspection are general precautions against electrical hazards. Specific precautions include the following[8]:

1. All instrument wiring in the blood bank should be approved by Underwriters Laboratories, or meet the requirements of the National Electric Code (NFPA 70), established by the National Fire Protection Association. All electrical installations, both fixed and portable, should conform to NFPA 70.[9]
2. All equipment must undergo periodic safety checks. These checks may be performed by blood bank staff or by facility engineering personnel; however, the safety status of each instrument should be indicated by a dated and initialed label or sticker placed on the instrument.
3. All defective electrical equipment should be tagged to warn employees of potential danger, and removed from service.
4. Do not overload outlets.
5. Do not remove or tamper with the grounding prong of a three-pronged plug, or use pigtail adapters. Pigtail adapters ground through the screw on the cover plate, but they cannot be assumed to be an adequate ground, and they may be disconnected inadvertently.
6. Do not use adapters that might allow equipment to be energized by voltages other than the design voltage.
7. Grounding circuits should be tested regularly to ensure that leakage currents are below safe minimums. Leakage currents from grounded equipment must be considerably lower if the instrument is to be attached to a human subject.[7] Testing services and information regarding current standards may be obtained from hospital-based biomedical engineers or from private contractors.

8. Electrical cords should never pass through door jambs. Protective covering on cords could easily be broken when the door is closed.
9. Do not extend electrical cords over or close to sinks.
10. Cords should be inspected periodically to ensure integrity of the insulation and contacts. Cords should be placed where they do not create trip hazards.
11. If cords are wired directly to equipment, they should be replaced by a qualified electrician.
12. Outlets should be located to minimize the need for extension cords.
13. Extension cords should not be used in place of permanent wiring.
14. Approved extension cords should be inspected regularly, and brittle or frayed cords should be replaced.
15. Do not run extension cords through walls, ceilings or doorways.
16. Extension outlet strips should be mounted whenever possible, and the power demand on an outlet strip should not exceed its maximum rating. Outlet strips should contain circuit breakers.
17. All electrical equipment should be turned off before connecting or disconnecting them from the power source.
18. Tools for working on electrical equipment should have insulated handles.
19. Use the "one hand rule," keeping one hand behind you, when working on electrical equipment.
20. Access to control switches, panels and circuit breakers should not be obstructed in any way. Outlets and switches should be labeled to indicate the panel location and circuit from which they are fed. Only qualified personnel should be allowed to reset circuit breakers.
21. Blood bank personnel should not work alone. They should be in sight of another employee who can call for assistance, who is familiar with the means of cutting off power, and with knowledge of emergency measures, such as fire extinguishers, cardiopulmonary resuscitation (CPR) and first aid.
22. All shocks, even very slight tingling sensations, from electrical equipment should be reported, and corrective actions should be taken.

In case of electrical shock, ask someone to call for assistance, and remove the source of shock as soon as possible. Using a dry towel or dry wooden pole, move the live wire or equipment away from the victim. If possible, turn off the power at the circuit breaker. Begin CPR immediately if necessary.

Mechanical Hazards

Broken glassware; obstructions such as supplies, carts, open drawers and doors, equipment or filing cabinets that impede traffic when improperly located in passageways; and improperly operated instruments such as centrifuges and autoclaves, are examples of mechanical hazards.

These hazards may produce injuries ranging from bruises and lacerations to serious injuries when parts of the body are caught, pinched or sheared. In addition, autoclave accidents may cause serious burns. Obstruction of aisles and passageways may impede evacuation in case of emergency.

Accidents caused by mechanical hazards may be substantially reduced through the following precautions:

1. Broken glassware should be discarded into containers provided for this purpose.
2. Aisles and passageways should be kept free of obstructions, and not used for storage. Drawers and cabinets should be kept closed.
3. Equipment should be operated according to the manufacturers' instructions.
4. Personnel should be thoroughly trained both in operating and troubleshooting procedures.
5. A program of preventive maintenance including function and safety checks should be developed and monitored.

The best sources of information regarding the prevention of accidents and injuries caused by specific hazards of blood bank instruments are the operator's manuals that accompany the instruments. These manuals and records of maintenance and repairs should be available at the bench for blood bank personnel.

Problems with the quality, performance or safety of a medical device or laboratory instrument may be reported to the Medical Device and Laboratory Product Problem Reporting Program, a program of the Department of Health and Human Services, Public Health Service, Food and Drug Administration, on forms provided by the program for that purpose.[10]

Although most accidents due to mechanical equipment hazards involve centrifuges or cell washers and autoclaves, other instruments found in the blood bank may present potential hazards to employees. Mechanical equipment becomes a safety hazard if it is located in such a way that the operator is exposed to traffic or constant interruptions. Also essential for accident prevention are the provision of adequate lighting and utilities; adequate space for maintenance and repairs; suitable waste containers; and storage of reagents, accessories, samples and manuals.

Autoclaves

Injuries caused by improper use of the autoclave include burns caused by very hot surfaces and steam, and injuries caused by objects propelled out of the autoclave during the rapid release of pressure. Employee training in the proper use of autoclaves is essential in protecting personnel from injuries. Other precautions include:
1. A summary of operating instructions should be posted near the autoclave, and the requirements for preparing materials to be autoclaved should be included.
2. Temperature and pressure settings should be appropriate for the materials to be autoclaved, and operators must check the settings and the indicator dials before they leave the vicinity of the instrument.
3. Before opening the autoclave, operators should make certain that the temperature and pressure have returned to normal levels.
4. Insulated gloves designed for this purpose should be used when placing items into, or removing them from the autoclave.

Centrifuges

Since centrifuges are capable of generating high speeds and considerable force, they have the potential to produce damage to property and injuries to employees. Larger instruments should be installed by the manufacturer.

All materials placed into the centrifuge should be sealed, capped or covered with parafilm to prevent contamination of the instrument and production of aerosols.

Rotors must be properly seated after cleaning or maintenance. If the holders are removable, they must be carefully replaced, and must rotate freely. The rotor must be free of debris and materials used for balance.

Materials to be centrifuged must be carefully balanced to prevent excessive vibration, which may cause severe damage to the instrument and anyone or anything near it.

Most new centrifuges are equipped with latches, which will prevent operation of the instrument unless the latches are secured. Centrifuges should not be operated with the covers open. The covers should not be unlatched until the rotor has stopped completely, and under no circumstances should personnel attempt to stop centrifuges with their hands.

Multichannel Automated Instruments

Operators should be equipped with safety glasses or goggles when changing tubing on any multichannel instrument.

Radiation Hazards

Radioactive Materials

Although the amount of radioactive material required to perform tests in the blood bank is usually small, some preventive measures and monitoring are appropriate. All procedures involving radioactive materials should be performed in compliance with the guidelines established by the radiation safety officer for the facility and the director of the laboratory.

Certain routine laboratory safety precautions need to be emphasized where procedures involving radioisotopes are performed[11]:

1. Frequent hand washing will minimize the possibility of unnecessary exposure to radiation.
2. Mechanical pipetting equipment should be provided to eliminate the need to pipette radioactive reagents by mouth.
3. Laboratory coats and disposable gloves should be worn whenever radioactive materials are being used.

In addition, there are several specific precautions that should be taken when handling radioactive materials:

1. All users of unsealed sources of radioactivity should cover bench tops with absorbant top, waterproof back bench-top covers to protect lab facilities from contamination whenever radioactive materials are used.
2. Radioactive spills should be reported to a supervisor, and cleaned up by an approved method.
3. To limit the amount of radioactive contamination in case of an accident, radioisotope procedures and equipment should be separated from other equipment and activities. The area should be clearly marked with a radiation sign. Laboratories

using radioactive materials should be locked when they are not occupied.

4. To monitor the amount of radiation exposure to personnel, safety film badges or ring monitors must be worn daily by anyone working with radioisotopes. The badges should be checked monthly, and the reports of the film readings should be recorded and monitored.

5. Laboratory work areas should be monitored for contamination by performing background counts (wipe-tested) monthly. The results should be recorded.

6. All used glassware, vials, contaminated towels, contaminated gloves, bench-top covers and radioactive materials should be placed in large yellow metal cans clearly labeled for the disposal of radioactive materials.

In case of accident such as possible body contamination, ingestion of radioactivity, overexposure, contamination of equipment, spread of contamination, difficulty in cleaning up a spill or loss of radioactive materials, notify the radiation safety officer or the laboratory director. Approved emergency cleanup and decontamination procedures should be written and available to the staff. All employees working with radioactive materials should be trained in these procedures.

Lasers

Radiation produced by lasers varies widely in type and intensity, depending on the design of the instrument. Lasers can produce burns and eye damage, and the following precautions apply[12,13]:

1. Do not look directly at the beam or the pump source.

2. Do not observe the beam pattern directly; use an indirect means such as an image converter. Do not aim by looking along the beam.

3. Do not allow reflective objects such as spherical buttons or polished screw heads to be present in or along the beam.

4. Maintain a high level of general illumination in the area. Low light levels allow pupil dilation, and increase the risk of eye injury.

5. Wear goggles to protect against the specific wavelength of the laser in use when working in areas in which the potential exposure to direct or reflected laser light greater than 0.005 watt exists. The goggles should be labeled with their effective wavelength protection, and separate goggles should be provided for each wavelength produced.[13]

6. Only qualified trained employees should operate laser equipment.
7. Areas in which lasers are being used shall be posted.
8. Beam shutters or caps should be used when the laser is not being used.
9. Laser equipment should be labeled to indicate maximum output.

Ultraviolet Light

Ultraviolet (UV) lamps produce two types of hazards: those produced by the radiation, and those caused by the use of the lamps.

The major biological effects of overexposure to ultraviolet radiation include irritation and damage to eye tissue, sunburn and skin cancer. Protective safety goggles with UV absorbing lenses should be worn when the eyes may be exposed to radiation with wavelengths shorter than 250 nm. Skin exposed to UV light can receive painful burns, so steps should be taken to protect the skin.

The second potential danger in using UV lamps is due to the buildup of UV absorbing residues on the inside of the mercury arc lamps. After a maximum number of hours of operation, these residues cause the temperature inside the lamp to rise above safe operating levels, and may cause the lamp to explode. Records should be kept of the number of hours of use. UV sources should be properly cooled, and completely enclosed to prevent injury due to flying glass fragments and the leakage of mercury vapor.[12,13]

Overexposure to UV radiation is usually indicated by reddening of the skin. In case of overexposure to UV radiation, report the incident and take appropriate corrective action. Obtain medical assistance if necessary.

Compressed Gases

Compressed gas cylinders may contain up to 3000 psi pressure. Improper handling of compressed gas cylinders may cause the release of gases with sufficient force to propel the cylinder through a wall, and produce significant injury and property damage.

Prevention of accidents caused by the mishandling of compressed gas cylinders depends on a few common sense rules[12-14]:

1. Compressed gas cylinders should be transported on wheeled carts to which they are securely fastened, and should always have the shipping caps on.
2. Gas cylinders should be labeled as to the contents. Double-check the label before connecting the cylinder. Unlabeled cylinders should not be used.
3. Cylinders should be stored and used in an upright position, and they should be fastened securely to a firm support.
4. The valves should not be opened with a hammer or a wrench. The valves, fittings and regulator should not be lubricated or tampered with.
5. Remove emptied cylinders from the laboratory promptly. The valves should be tightly closed, and the cylinders should be handled carefully, since they should contain more than 100 psi of positive pressure to prevent contamination of the cylinders when they are "empty."
6. Use the smallest sized compressed gas cylinder appropriate for the purpose. Do not store cylinders in the laboratory.
7. The cylinders should never be stored or used near a source of heat.

Cryogenic Liquids

Cryogenic liquids and their gases and surfaces represent a serious hazard to living tissue in the form of frostbite or actual freezing. The hazard is comparable to that of boiling water or live steam. Furthermore, cryogenic liquids exhibit a volume change ratio of about 1:700 to over 1:1000 on vaporization, which can cause rapid, violent pressure changes. Rupturing or even explosion of a vessel can result if the valve becomes plugged with water or ice.

Cryogenic liquids have boiling points from about -100 to -270 C. All of them are liquified under pressure and frequently used at atmospheric pressure. Thus, they are constantly boiling during use.

Cryogenic liquids and compressed gases have many properties in common; hence, they have many hazards in common, including: low boiling point, pressure, some support combustion and rapid diffusion. Many of the rules for the storage and handling of compressed gases apply to cryogenic liquids.

Most materials subjected to cryogenic temperatures (-100 to -270 C) experience some degree of embrittlement. Living tissue can become so brittle that it will shatter. Cryogenic liquids should not be allowed to contact any materials not designed for use in that particular procedure. Select working materials carefully, since cryogenic temperatures may alter the physical characteristics of many materials.

Liquid nitrogen can condense liquid oxygen from the atmosphere, causing an explosion if any organic material is also condensed. All cryogens can condense sufficient moisture from the air to block the opening in storage vessels. An explosion can result due to pressure buildup. Avoid contact of moisture with storage containers to prevent ice plugging of relief devices. Keep all systems clean.

All cryogenic liquids also produce large volumes of gas when they vaporize, which can displace the air in an area where they are in use. If these liquids are vaporized in a sealed container, they can produce enormous pressures. For this reason, pressurized cryogenic containers are usually provided with multiple pressure relief devices. Use only approved storage and transport vessels, which have pressure relief fittings. Store and use cryogenic liquids in well-ventilated areas to prevent displacement of air.[8]

Personnel handling cryogenic liquids need to be informed of the hazards, and trained to handle these materials in a safe manner[8]:

1. Eye protection should be required during transfer and normal handling of cryogens. Face shields may be advisable if the operation may result in splashing or spraying of the cryogen.
2. Dry leather gloves that are loose fitting (so that they can be removed quickly if liquids are spilled into them) or pot holders should be used whenever handling anything that comes in contact with cryogenic liquids or vapor.
3. Depending on the application, special clothing may be required.

For short contact or exposure, flush the area with large quantities of water (high heat capacity). Get medical attention. For any exposure that is prolonged, or if visible tissue damage is apparent, immediate medical attention is needed to restore tissues to normal temperature.[8]

Flammables and Fire Hazards

The process of burning, or the rapid oxidation of a fuel by an oxidizer with the liberation of heat and light, involves three interrelated components: fuel, oxidizer and ignition source. For a fire to occur, all three components must be present.

For practical purposes, the fuel and the oxidizer, usually air, must be present in sufficient quantity to form an ignitable mixture, and the ignition source, containing sufficient energy to initiate combustion, must be present. The ignition source may be in the form of a spark, flame or heat alone. A fire can start only when sufficient energy is present to initiate and sustain the chemical reaction, and when the fuel and oxidizer are present in optimal proportions.

Preventing fires is a matter of eliminating the oxidizer, the fuel or the ignition source. Since air is usually the oxidizer, removing this component would prevent a fire from starting, but the environment and oxygen sources are relatively difficult to control. A successful fire prevention program must focus on understanding the properties of flammable and combustible materials present in the blood bank, controlling their use and removing all possible sources of ignition.

Fires are classified into four groups (Classes A, B, C and D) according to the nature of the combustible material. These classes, which were developed by the Underwriters Laboratories and adopted by the National Fire Protection Association,[15] are defined as follows:

Class A includes fires of ordinary materials present in the laboratory such as wood, plastics, paper and textiles, ie, elements that require the quenching and cooling action of water or water-based solutions for their extinguishment.

Class B includes fires of flammable liquids and gases, ie, elements that require the exclusion of oxygen from the source of fuel for their extinguishment.

Class C includes fires in energized electrical equipment, which require for their extinguishment the use of nonconductive media.

Class D includes fires of combustible and reactive chemicals such as sodium, potassium, magnesium and lithium. These fires pose special problems of control and extinguishment, since spreading and explosion can easily occur.

Fire Prevention

Flammable solvents are one of the most common sources of fires. A flammable solvent is an organic liquid whose vapor can form an ignitable mixture with air, and whose flash point, or the minimum temperature at which sufficient vapors are produced to form an ignitable mixture with the air near the surface of the liquid, is less than 100 C.

The storage of flammable and combustible liquids in a laboratory must be kept to the minimum needed for research or operations. The following precautions should be observed whenever flammable liquids are used[16]:

1. Store flammable solvents in areas that are well-ventilated (to prevent buildup of vapors) and free of ignition sources.
2. When using or dispensing flammable solvents, use a working fume hood with a velocity of at least 100 ft/min. Whenever possible, work with flammables 10-12 C below the flash point.
3. Use safety cans for storage and transfer of flammables. Keep all cans, drums and other containers tightly closed. If more than 5 gal of flammable liquids in glass must be stored per 100 sq ft of laboratory space, an approved flammables safety cabinet must be provided.
4. Label containers into which flammables are transferred with all precautionary information.
5. Do not work with flammables near a source of ignition.
6. Do not store flammables in glass on shelves above counter level.
7. Use explosion-proof refrigerators for flammables that need refrigeration, even if stored temporarily.

Storage cabinets are designed and constructed to limit the internal temperature to not more than 325 F when subjected to a 10-minute fire test using the standard time/temperature chart set forth by the NFPA. Flammable safety cabinets should be labeled "Flammable—Keep Fire Away." Approved flammables cabinets are constructed of at least 18-gauge sheet iron and should be double-walled with 1½ inch air space. Joints should be riveted, welded or made tight by some equally effective means. The door should be provided with a three point lock, and the door sill should be raised at least two inches above the bottom of the cabinet. All flammables cabinets must be grounded using a ground cable of 3/8 inch copper braid or 12-gauge copper conductor. The ground should be tested, and the resistance to ground cannot exceed one megohm. The grounding cable must be connected to a building structural member or a building electrical ground. Due to the increased use of plastic piping, water pipes should no longer be used for grounding.[8]

The NFPA Technical Committee on General Storage of Flammable Liquids considers that providing vents to storage cabinets reduces the limited fire protection provided by such cabinets because a single-walled duct will transmit heat faster than a double-walled cabinet. Ventilation of storage cabinets is recommended only where required by local ordinance, or where highly odiferous conditions exist. Ventilation requires a steel duct and an appropriate exhaust fan discharging to a safe location.[8]

No more than 60 gallons of Class I flammable liquids (flash point below 100 F) or Class II combustible liquids (flash point between 100 F and 140 F) may be stored in a flammables storage cabinet. All chemicals stored in a flammables cabinet must be compatible.[8]

Disposal of flammable liquids into the sewage system should be prohibited. The exceptions include flammable liquids that are miscible with water. These may be disposed of through the sewage system provided the volume does not exceed one pint, and the flammable liquids are mixed with large quantities of cold water. Refer to local and Environmental Protection Agency (EPA) regulations. Most flammables must be disposed of in safety cans or metal drums designed for this purpose.[17]

Another fire hazard in the laboratory is the storage of combustible materials, especially records. Good housekeeping is essential in storage areas. Combustibles should never be stored in the same area with flammables, nor should they be stored in areas not protected by sprinklers.

Fire Fighting

The key elements in effective fire fighting include: fire detection systems and properly located employee alarm systems, adequate numbers of well-maintained fire extinguishers and fire blankets, well-marked exits free of obstructions and thorough employee training and rehearsal of fire fighting procedures.

Heat and smoke detectors should be located throughout the facility, including storage areas. Alarm systems should be located such that all employees are dependably warned of possible fires. Sprinklers should also be present in areas where there is the risk of fire. Halon systems should be considered instead of sprinklers in areas used to house computers. Consult with the hardware vendor for the recommended method of fire extinguishment.

Occupational Safety and Health Administration (OSHA) standards require that employers provide appropriate fire extinguishing systems in the work place.[18] Automatic sprinkler systems, fixed extinguisher systems or portable fire extinguishers are acceptable. If the laboratory Emergency Action Plan calls for the total evacuation of all employees in case of fire, portable fire fighting equipment is not required. However, if portable fire extinguishers are provided, it is the employer's responsibility to ensure their proper maintenance, inspection and distribution. Portable fire extinguishers should be mounted on the wall, no more than 5 feet from the ground so that they can be removed without subjecting employees to the possibility of injury.[19]

The concentrations of Halon and carbon dioxide used in fixed extinguishing systems are limited by OSHA regulations depending on the time employees may be exposed. Fire extinguishing chemicals may be hazardous to employees because of their concentrations, or because of toxic decomposition products formed when the fire fighting agents come in contact with hot surfaces. High expansion foam agents may interfere with breathing and vision, although they are not normally toxic. Foam extinguishing systems available in the laboratory must conform with NFPA standards for the installation of such systems.[20,21]

Safety Equipment

For convenience, this discussion of safety equipment has been divided into two categories:
1. Personal protective equipment used routinely for protection against known or anticipated hazards.
2. Emergency equipment used for the protection of life and property in the event of an accident.

Personal Protective Equipment

Part of management's responsibility in an effective safety program is to provide any personal protective equipment required to handle safely any hazard found in the blood bank. Policies for the blood bank should include the requirement for protective equipment for appropriate procedures, and all personnel should be trained in their proper use during the orientation period.

Safety Glasses or Goggles

Eye protection should be worn whenever procedures are being performed that could result in splashing of liquid nitrogen, serum, reagents or other potentially harmful substances into the eyes; for example, in the freezing of red cells units or droplets, and leukocytes and when changing the tubing on an automated blood typing instrument.

Laboratory Coats

Laboratory coats or aprons afford some protection against risk of infection from serum, burns due to liquid nitrogen and dry ice and injury due to flying glass. However, there are some conditions that must be met in order to maximize the benefit to employees:
1. Coats should be worn buttoned or snapped closed, and should allow for quick exit in case of a spill.
2. Remove laboratory coats worn at the bench before leaving the laboratory; do not wear them to the cafeteria or in patient areas.
3. Do not launder clothing worn in the laboratory with domestic articles of clothing.

Disposable Gloves

Disposable gloves may be used whenever specimens of known or undetermined hazard must be handled. The need for gloves should be evaluated by each laboratory based on an assessment of the risk. Employees with cuts on their hands should work in gloves; however, gloves must be removed before leaving the laboratory. The gloves should be removed at the bench or in the patient's room immediately after completing the procedure, and disposed of properly. Gloves should not be worn to answer the telephone, or to perform other tasks during an incubation phase.

Emergency Equipment

When emergency equipment is required, time is critical. The type and location of emergency equipment should be carefully planned and appropriate for the types of emergencies that could be expected to occur. All employees must know the exact location and function of all emergency equipment within the area. All employees must be trained in the use of emergency equipment in the blood bank. Certain types of emergency equipment, such as oxygen masks, should be used only by specially trained individuals, and should be labeled "To be used by trained personnel only."

Eyewash Fountains and Safety Showers

If corrosive materials are in use, suitable facilities for rapid, thorough flushing of the eyes and body should be provided within 25 feet of the work area available for immediate use. Valve handles should be rigidly fixed and clearly labeled. Chain pulls should have large rings. The water supply for the showers should be of drinking quality. These systems must be inspected periodically, and tagged with the results of these inspections. All employees must be trained in the proper use of the eyewash stations and safety showers.[8,12,13]

In case of a chemical spill that contacts clothing or skin, remove affected clothing immediately, and rinse with large quantities of cold water for at least 15 minutes. Do not attempt to wash off with solvents, bleach, alkali or other chemical solutions. All spills should be reported.

Eyewash fountains should provide a gentle stream of temperate, aerated water for at least 15 minutes. Hands should not be necessary to maintain water flow. The eyewash fountains should be inspected regularly, and a record of the inspections should be maintained. All personnel should be trained in their use. If possible, the eyewash fountains should be located adjacent to the safety showers so that the eyes can be washed at the same time that the rest of the body is being showered.[8,12,13]

In case of chemical splashes, an immediate 15-minute irrigation is indicated with copious amounts of water under gentle pressure. Check for and remove contact lenses quickly, but do not delay washing if the lenses are difficult to remove. Hold the eye open to wash under the eyelid and rotate the eye so that all surfaces of the eye are rinsed. Cover the eyes with clean, wet, soft pads and obtain prompt medical attention.[13]

Spill Kits

Spill kits are available in a variety of sizes and types, for both biohazard spills and chemical spills. These spill kits should be readily accessible, and all employees should be trained in their use. Once the kit has been used, it should be replaced immediately.

In case of a spill that is not volatile or toxic, and where no fire hazard exists, clean up the spill using an absorbent material that will neutralize it. Wear gloves, and use a dust pan and brush to pick up the neutralized absorbed material. Dispose of the material in the appropriate solid waste container. Do not leave paper towels and absorbents used to clean up a spill in open trash cans in the work area. Following neutralization and clean up, clean the area with soap and water and mop dry or spread more of the absorbent to prevent slipping.[5]

If a volatile, flammable, or toxic material is spilled, warn other employees in the area to extinguish flames, turn off all equipment (especially instruments with brush type motors) and vacate the room until the spill has been cleaned up. Report all spills immediately. A supervisor should determine the extent of evacuation and the cleanup procedure.[13]

First Aid Kit

First aid kits should be provided in all work areas, and should be stocked with items needed for the types of accidents that could be expected to occur. Instructions for the use of the first aid supplies should be posted near or in the kit, and should be included in the safety manual. Following first aid, injured persons should report for further medical evaluation and treatment, accompanied by another person knowledgeable about the accident.

All blood bank staff should be trained in basic first aid, and personnel trained in cardiopulmonary resuscitation (CPR) should be immediately available, especially when donor procedures are performed.

Fire Alarms

Every facility should develop emergency procedures that include properly located smoke and heat detection devices, and that provide for fire alarm activation. All employees must be instructed in the proper procedure for reporting a fire, and all workers should know the locations of the fire alarm boxes in their areas.

Building Emergency Alarms

If an alarm system is used to warn employees of fire or other facility emergencies, the codes and instructions must be prominently posted in every room in the facility. The alarms should be tested frequently, and there should be a backup alarm system in addition to the telephones.

Fire Extinguishers

The proper type, number and placement of fire extinguishers is another essential feature of an effective fire fighting program. Each of the four classes of fires requires a different means of extinguishment depending upon the nature of the combustible material[19]:

Class A extinguishers are used on Class A fires and include foam, loaded stream and multipurpose dry chemical extinguishers. A number preceding the class rating indicates the relative effectiveness of the fire extinguisher.

Class B extinguishers are used on Class B fires, and include bromotrifluoromethane (Halon 1301), bromochlorodifluoromethane (Halon 1211), carbon dioxide, dry chemical, foam and loaded stream extinguishers.

Class C extinguishers are used on Class C fires and include bromotrifluoromethane, bromochorodifluoromethane, carbon dioxide and dry chemical extinguishers.

Class D extinguishers are used on Class D fires and contain dry powder media, which do not react or combine adversely with the burning materials.

The number and class rating of the extinguishers selected should correspond to the hazards present in the laboratory. In general, the higher the rating the larger the area that can be protected by the extinguisher. The maximum recommended travel distance to Class A fire extinguishers is 75 feet.[22] Class B extinguishers are also rated for maximum travel distance to the extinguisher and for the area to be protected.

Extinguishers for Class C fires should be located in areas where energized electrical equipment is being used. The extinguishing media for Class C extinguishers is a nonconductive material. De-energized electrical equipment fires can be extinguished with Class A or B extinguishers. Class C extinguishers should be located as recommended for Class B extinguishers, ie, 30-50 feet maximum travel distance depending on the hazard.[19]

There would be little application for Class D fire extinguishers in the blood bank.

Personnel who are expected to use the fire extinguishers must be thoroughly trained to operate fire fighting equipment effectively and to understand the properties of the chemicals used in the fire extinguishers. In addition, all prospective users must be familiar with the location and type of extinguishers in their areas.

Extinguishers used in the blood bank must be selected according to the class and extent of the fire hazard and the rating of the extinguisher. Some of the extinguishing chemicals pose a low toxicity hazard to the employees. There may be a more serious hazard produced by the accumulation of the agent or of its decomposition products. For example, the use of a carbon dioxide extinguisher in a small area may result in a depletion of oxygen.

Extinguishers should be inspected at least once a month. Access to extinguishers should not be blocked, and they should not be used for door stops. Extinguishers should be replaced immediately after use. The manufacturer's recommended maintenance procedures should be performed annually, and the extinguishers tagged with the record of the inspection.

Emergency Exits

Emergency exits should be clearly marked and readily accessible at all times. They should never be chained or locked, and should never be obstructed.

Evacuation Plan

Each facility should develop an evacuation plan and post it in conspicuous places. The plan should contain at least the following:
1. The procedure for notification. Keys for bell codes or public address system codes should be included. An adequate primary and backup communication system should be available, in addition to the telephone.
2. Floor plan with evacuation routes indicated. Several alternative routes should be included.
3. Instructions to turn off specific instruments, close the doors and to use the stairwells instead of the elevators.
4. Instructions to proceed to a meeting point outside the building, and not to return to the building until told to do so by an authorized person.

In addition, the plan should specify a staff member who is designated to make a complete check of the area to make sure everyone is out of the building. The plan should also provide for assistance from outside emergency services such as the police and fire departments, emergency services, public utilities and a nearby hospital. Crews to handle first aid, fire fighting, searches, engineering problems and chemical or biohazard spills need to be developed and trained.

Evacuations should be rehearsed periodically, the posted information updated, evacuation routes checked and reports kept of these rehearsals. Documentation of corrective actions should be maintained.

Fire Drills

A schedule of fire drills should be the responsibility of a safety officer or safety committee. Fire drill procedures should be written, available to all employees in their procedures manuals and part of the employee orientation program.

Drills should be held periodically, including during off-hour shifts, and the performance of all concerned should be observed. These observations and any corrective actions should be documented.

The Role of Management

Facility Planning

A safe working environment is more than simply making all employees more aware and more careful; it requires planning and preparation. For management, this requires design of the laboratories and selection of equipment to ensure proper space, light, storage, ventilation, appropriate disposal of waste and immediate access to appropriate safety equipment.

The Building

The National Fire Protection Association recommends that hospital laboratories be separated from other hospital areas and from exit corridors by fire resistant construction of at least 1-hour rating. Subdivisions of the laboratory should also be separated from each other by 1-hour, fire resistant construction.[23] Single laboratory units should not exceed 5000 sq ft.

There are standards for interior paint that should be used in the laboratories, in access corridors and in routes to exits to limit the spread of flames. Metal cabinets, benches and shelving are the furniture of choice. Furniture made of other materials should have fire retardant finishes. Wall cabinets should be securely anchored and soffits should be used to prevent overloading on the top of cabinets.[23]

The surfaces of counter tops and floors should be covered with impervious materials that facilitate decontamination and cleaning. The counter tops should curve smoothly into a rear splash panel at least 6 inches high.

A valuable reference for fireproofing is the National Fire Code of the National Fire Protection Association. Local construction codes are another useful source of information, as are insurance industry standards.

There should be adequate numbers of exits in each area, depending on the size and function of the area. Exits should have outward swing doors. See the American Standards Association Exit Code for details. Aisles in laboratory work areas should be wide enough to allow rapid exit in case of emergency, and to avoid crowding of personnel performing routine functions. The minimum width for single aisles is 36 inches; for double aisles between island benches it is 60 inches.[23]

Lighting sources of 100 foot-candles should be provided, properly secured and arranged so as to reduce shadowing. Guards should not be broken or missing. Electrical panels should be located immediately adjacent to the laboratory. Emergency power should be sufficient to maintain essential services.[23]

Sinks and drains should be properly placed, and should be made of materials that are resistant to chemicals customarily used in the facility. Consideration should be given to installing clinical sinks in areas where local ordinances permit disposal of blood samples into the drains.

The National Electrical Code of the National Fire Prevention Association is a good reference for electrical specifications. Use only three-prong convenience outlets. Do not locate outlets near sinks or other grounded equipment. An independent building ground is required. Water pipes should not be used as grounds.[8]

Arrangement

There are two popular types of laboratory arrangements: those with peninsula-type benches and those with island-type benches. The island arrangement has the advantage that there are no barriers to emergency exits.

Locate hoods away from exits in order to prevent blocking of the exits in case of accident in the hood. Hoods should be located away from desks and offices.

Office areas should be remote from the laboratory areas when possible. At least, plan for partitions or safety shields to separate laboratory areas from office areas.

If the degree of hazard warrants, locate a safety shower near the exit in the room where the hazard exits. Showers should have deluge-type heads and the controls should be quick-opening.

Eyewash stations should be provided in every hazardous location, preferably near an exit.

Fire extinguishers for every type of fire that can occur in a given location should be provided. Safety shields, fire blankets, safety goggles and spill cleanup kits should be immediately available in the laboratory.

Electrical outlets should be adequately grounded, and not located near sinks, other grounded equipment or in the hoods.

Storage Facilities

Central storage facilities reduce the individual storage area needed in laboratories. Stock of common equipment can be maintained. Equipment and records storage should be separate from reagent storerooms. A separate storage area should be available for flammables.

Storeroom shelves that can be accessed from both sides should have partitions in the center or high sills. Earthquake bars should be installed on shelves in earthquake prone areas. Drawers should have stops to prevent drawers from being pulled out of the guides.

Safety cabinets with adequate ventilation should be provided for stored chemicals, especially flammables. Chemical storage should be arranged so that reactive chemicals can be isolated from each other. Separate oxidizers, corrosives, flammables and toxicants. For flammable materials requiring refrigeration, use only a refrigerator with an explosion-proof interior.

Do not store excess reagents, flammables or obsolete equipment.

A Safety Program

Develop a safety program in the laboratory or in the facility based on the philosophy that accidents can be prevented, and include the following:

1. Write a safety manual. Require all technical, clerical and administrative personnel; students; and new employees to read it and sign a statement that they have done so, and that they understand the contents.
2. Develop a safety orientation program for new employees.

3. Organize a safety committee or safety audit team, and have them meet regularly to discuss and resolve safety problems.
4. Conduct periodic, unannounced safety inspections to find and correct hazardous conditions and unsafe practices.
5. Schedule regular departmental safety meetings to discuss the results of safety inspections or aspects of blood bank safety. These sessions should be an integral part of staff continuing education.
6. Require that all accidents or incidents be reported to and evaluated by the safety committee, and discussed at the departmental safety meetings.
7. Develop plans and conduct drills for dealing with emergencies such as fire, explosion, injury to an employee or donor or a severe donor reaction.
8. Display the phone numbers of the fire department, police or security department, ambulance or emergency services and the engineering department immediately next to every telephone.
9. Post warning signs in areas involving radioactivity, lasers, biological hazards or other special hazards.
10. Require good housekeeping practices in all work areas.
11. Maintain an inventory of chemicals such that the supply of chemicals on hand at one time is kept to a minimum. Label all chemicals to show the nature and degree of hazard, and necessary precautions for handling.
12. Develop a system for the safe and ecologically acceptable disposal of chemical wastes. The system should specify a method for dating stored chemicals and for discarding materials after the expiration date.
13. Allocate a portion of the budget for safety.
14. Provide adequate safety equipment—personal protective equipment, emergency equipment and first aid supplies— and require that every employee be trained to use safety equipment. Inspect and maintain safety equipment on a regular basis.
15. Maintain a centrally located, easily accessible safety library, which could contain some of the references listed in Appedix 2-1.

Safety Audit

A safety audit, or work place hazard analysis, should be conducted on a regular basis. The purpose of the audit is to prevent accidents by identifying the hazards, reporting them, recommending corrective actions and providing persistent followup.

A safety committee or safety audit team consisting of concerned supervisors, and if possible, a representative from the facility safety department should be formed. In addition to routine inspections, the responsibilities of the safety audit team might include review of accidents or incidents, and coordination of safety training.

The goal of the audit team is to identify the hazards in the following major areas: housekeeping, mechanical, chemical, thermal, electrical, pressure, safety equipment and training.

The first step in a safety audit is to review the accident history and the previous safety inspection reports for the facility. Some sources of information include accident reports, safety inspection reports and inspection reports of accreditation agencies. Summarize the significant hazards, especially repeat problems. Evaluate previous efforts to correct the hazards.

The second step is the inspection itself. Involve the supervisor in the inspection. Use a checklist and issue a report of the inspection promptly. Appendix 2-2 contains an example of a safety checklist, which may be adapted to your facility.

Summary

Prevention of accidents through the development and implementation of an effective safety program depends on the identification of any hazards present in the facility, the consistent application of appropriate precautions, the availability of safety equipment, clearly defined emergency policies and procedures, training and retraining of all employees and continuous monitoring of the safety status of the facility.

References

1. Widmann FK, ed. Technical manual. 9th ed. Arlington, VA: American Association of Blood Banks, 1985.
2. Inspection checklist. Laboratory general. Skokie, IL: College of American Pathologists, Commission on Laboratory Accreditation, 1985.
3. Accreditation manual for hospitals. Chicago, IL: Joint Commission on Hospital Accreditation, 1987.
4. Association for Practitioners in Infection Control. New Jersey task force report on safe needle and syringe disposal. Princeton, NJ: Association for Practitioners in Infection Control, New Jersey Hospital Association, 1985.

5. State of New Jersey P.L. 1985 C96 (2A:170-35.17). Trenton, NJ: State of New Jersey, 1985.
6. Garza D, Becan-McBride K. Phlebotomy handbook. New York: Appleton-Century-Crofts, 1984.
7. Steere NV. Physical, chemical, and fire safety. In: Fuscaldo AA, Erlick BJ, Hindman B, eds. Laboratory safety: theory and practice. New York: Academic Press, 1980.
8. JT Baker Chemical Company. Environmental health and safety. 4th ed. JT Baker Chemical Company, 1986.
9. National Fire Protection Association. National electric codes. Vol 5 national fire codes. Boston, MA: National Fire Protection Association, 1986.
10. Department of Health and Human Services, Public Health Service, Food and Drug Administration. Medical device and laboratory product problem reporting program form. Rockville, MD: Food and Drug Administration, 1984.
11. Radiation safety policy manual. Newark, NJ: University of Medicine and Dentistry of New Jersey, 1979.
12. Safety and health manual. Salt Lake City, UT: University of Utah, Department of Public Safety, 1982.
13. Safety in academic chemistry laboratories. 4th ed. Washington, DC: American Chemical Society, 1985.
14. National Safety Council. Safety for supervisors. 5th ed. Chicago, IL: National Safety Council, 1980.
15. National Fire Protection Association. Fire protection handbook. NFPA No. 1. Boston, MA: National Fire Protection Association, 1975.
16. Moya CE, Guarda LA, Sodeman TM. Safety in the clinical laboratory. Part 3: flammable solvents. Lab Med 1980;11(9): 582-4.
17. National Fire Protection Association. Safety standards for laboratories in health related institutions. NFPA No. 56A. Boston, MA: National Fire Protection Association, 1973.
18. Occupational Safety and Health Administration. Means of egress, hazardous materials, and fire protection. Rockville, MD: US Department of Labor, Occupational Safety and Health Administration, 1978.
19. Moya CE, Guarda LA, Sodeman TM. Safety in the clinical laboratory. Part 2: fire protection, prevention, and control. Lab Med 1980;11(9):578-81.
20. National Fire Protection Association. Standard for foam extinguishing systems. NFPA No. 11. Boston, MA: National Fire Protection Association, 1978.
21. National Fire Protection Association. Standard for high expansion foam systems (expansion ratios from 1:100 to

1:1000). NFPA No. 11a. Boston, MA: National Fire Protection Association, 1976.

22. National Fire Protection Association. Standard for portable fire extinguishers. NFPA No. 10. Boston, MA: National Fire Protection Association, 1978.

23. Bond RG, Michaelsen GS, DeRoos RL. Environmental health and safety in health care facilities. New York: Macmillan Publishing Co. Inc., 1973.

Appendix 2-1. References in a Safety Library

Alphabetical Index of Industrial Data Sheets
National Safety Council
425 North Michigan Ave.
Chicago, IL 60611

The Merck Index: An Encyclopedia of Chemicals and Drugs
Merck and Company, Inc.
126 East Lincoln Ave.
Rahway, NJ 07065

Safety in Academic Laboratories (1 copy free)
American Chemical Society
1155 16th St. NW
Washington, DC 20036

Fire Protection Guide on Hazardous Materials ($10)
National Fire Protection Association
Batterymarch Park
Quincy, MA 02269

Handbook of Laboratory Safety ($60)
Edited by N. Steere
CRC Press
2000 Corporate Blvd, NW
Boca Raton, FL 33431

Laboratory Safety Manual
Centers for Disease Control
Atlanta, Ga 30333

Safety Standard for Laboratories in Health Related Institutions
NFPA Publ. No.56C
National Fire Protection Association
Batterymench Park
Quincy, MA 02269

Dangerous Properties of Industrial Materials
Edited by N.I. Sax
Van Nostrand Reinhold Co.
135 W. 50th St.
New York, NY 10020

Prudent Practices for Handling Chemicals in Laboratories ($15)
Prudent Practices for Disposal of Chemicals from Laboratories
($15)
National Academy Press
2101 Constitution Ave. NW
Washington, DC 20418

(The following are available from the Superintendent of
Documents, US Printing Office, Washington, DC 20402)

Registry of Toxic Effects of Chemical Substances
US Dept. of Health and Human Services
Public Health Service

Occupational Health Guidelines
NIOSH/OSHA (NIOSH Publ. No. 81-123)

NIOSH/OSHA Pocket Guide to Chemical Hazards
NIOSH Publ. No. 78-210

Appendix 2-2. Safety Checklist

Instructions:

1. Record observations during the inspection.

_____
Location

2. Designate serious hazards with an X, less serious hazards with a check in the requires action column.

_____
Inspected by

3. Give a copy to the supervisor.

4. Supervisor records the corrective action and date, and returns a copy to the safety audit team.

_____
Date

	Satisfactory	Requires Action	Action Taken	Date/by
1. *Housekeeping*				
1.1 Orderly working conditions. No crowding.	_____	_____	_____	_____
1.2 No unstable storage on shelves, cabinets or high places.	_____	_____	_____	_____
1.3 Arrangement of equipment and furniture allows unobstructed egress. Aisle width 36 inches. Aisles and corridors unobstructed.	_____	_____	_____	_____
1.4 Floors clean and dry.	_____	_____	_____	_____
1.5 No trip hazards.	_____	_____	_____	_____
1.6 Furniture and equipment secured against tipping and falling.	_____	_____	_____	_____
1.7 No food or beverages used or stored.	_____	_____	_____	_____
1.8 No smoking signs posted.	_____	_____	_____	_____
1.9 No sharp or protruding objects, open drawers or cabinets.	_____	_____	_____	_____
1.10 Furniture and equipment in good repair.	_____	_____	_____	_____
1.11 Appropriate storage and disposal containers for paper, broken glass, hazardous materials, and needles and syringes.	_____	_____	_____	_____
1.12 Lighting sufficient.	_____	_____	_____	_____
1.13 No hood sashes open or hood obstructed.	_____	_____	_____	_____

	Satisfactory	Requires Action	Action Taken	Date/by
1.14 Storage outside of cabinets or storerooms kept to a minimum.	_____	_____	_____	_____
1.15 Adequate posting of hazardous areas.	_____	_____	_____	_____
2. Mechanical/Equipment				
2.1 Equipment maintenance.	_____	_____	_____	_____
2.2 Condition of equipment.	_____	_____	_____	_____
2.3 Adequate exhaust for fume hoods. Inspected annually.	_____	_____	_____	_____
2.4 Electrical/safety checks documented.	_____	_____	_____	_____
2.5 Location of equipment.	_____	_____	_____	_____
3. Electrical				
3.1 Equipment grounded, inspected.	_____	_____	_____	_____
3.2 Proper use of outlets.	_____	_____	_____	_____
3.3 Proper use of extension cords.	_____	_____	_____	_____
3.4 Unobstructed access to circuit breakers.	_____	_____	_____	_____
3.5 Properly installed plugs, cords and outlets. Maintained in good condition.	_____	_____	_____	_____
3.6 Cords kept away from sinks.	_____	_____	_____	_____
4. Chemical				
4.1 No excessive storage of chemicals.	_____	_____	_____	_____
4.2 Chemical labeling.	_____	_____	_____	_____
4.3 Safe storage of corrosive, flammable or toxic chemicals.	_____	_____	_____	_____
a. Safety cans and cabinets	_____	_____	_____	_____
b. Small volumes	_____	_____	_____	_____
c. Separation of incompatible chemicals	_____	_____	_____	_____
4.4 Materials data safety sheets available.	_____	_____	_____	_____
5. Compressed Gases				
5.1 Compressed gas cylinders secured.	_____	_____	_____	_____
5.2 Cylinder caps in place when not in use.	_____	_____	_____	_____
5.3 No laboratory storage of cylinders.	_____	_____	_____	_____
5.4 Cylinders labeled.	_____	_____	_____	_____

	Satisfactory	Requires Action	Action Taken	Date/by

6. Needles/Sharps
   6.1 Secure storage.
   6.2 Proper handling and
       disposal.

7. Fire Safety
   7.1 Tagging and removal of
       defective equipment.
   7.2 Adequate storage of
       combustibles.
   7.3 Adequate fire detection, and
       warning systems.
   7.4 Adequate fire fighting
       equipment.
   7.5 Well-marked, unobstructed
       exits.
   7.6 Proper storage of
       flammables.
   7.7 No Smoking signs posted
       and enforced.

8. Safety Equipment
   8.1 Fire extinguishers, blankets
       properly located, inspected
       and tagged.
   8.2 Safety showers and eyewash
       fountains accessible,
       inspected and tagged.
   8.3 Safety goggles or face
       shields available where
       appropriate.
   8.4 Laboratory coats worn.
   8.5 Disposable gloves available;
       used and discarded properly.
   8.6 Emergency exits marked.
   8.7 Evacuation plan posted in
       every room.
   8.8 Emergency numbers posted
       near every telephone.

9. Personnel
   9.1 Knowledge of fire alarms and
       evacuation procedure.
   9.2 Knowledge of safety rules.
   9.3 Adequate eye protection.
   9.4 Adequate personal protective
       equipment used.
   9.5 Regular safety training.
   9.6 Safety manual acknowledged
       by all employees.

	Satisfactory	Requires Action	Action Taken	Date/by
10. *Special Hazards*				
10.1 Special procedures implemented for:	_____	_____	_____	_____
a. Radiation sources	_____	_____	_____	_____
b. Cryogenic liquids	_____	_____	_____	_____
c. Lasers	_____	_____	_____	_____
d. UV light sources	_____	_____	_____	_____
10.2 Monitoring systems implemented, tested and functioning properly.	_____	_____	_____	_____

In: Gibbs, FL and Kasprisin, CA, eds.
Environmental Safety in the Blood Bank
Arlington, VA: American Association
of Blood Banks, 1987

3

Chemical Hazards in the Immunohematology Laboratory

Gerald A. Hoeltge, MD

*T*HE BLOOD BANKING LABORATORY has fewer serious chemical hazards in it than does the average chemistry or research laboratory. For this reason some immunohematologists have never become familiar with the standard precautionary terms for chemicals, practices for safe handling and storage or resources available for hazard containment and management of risk. Introduction of new laboratory technologies often implies the use of new chemicals. Every unfamiliar chemical must be researched before it can be introduced safely into routine practice. Moreover, some of the standard chemicals that have been in use in many blood banking laboratories for years are significantly hazardous. A general overview of the types of chemical hazards that are found in clinical laboratories follows to provide a context for the study of chemical hazards in immunohematology practice.

Classification of Chemical Hazards

Corrosives

The Environmental Protection Agency (EPA) has defined corrosive wastes on the basis of pH or the ability to corrode steel. Any aqueous waste that has a pH less than 2.1 or greater than 12.5, or a liquid waste that can corrode SAE 1020 steel more than 0.250 inch/year at 55 C is corrosive.[1,2] As a warning on a reagent label, however, the term may be used to refer to any substance that can cause visible destruction or irreversible alteration in human tissues at the site of contact.

Gerald A. Hoeltge, MD, Chairman, Department of Blood Banking, The Cleveland Clinic Foundation, Cleveland, Ohio

Asphyxiants

Asphyxiants are those chemicals that exert an adverse effect by displacing atmospheric oxygen or by prohibiting metabolic use of available oxygen. Many gases can be asphyxiating in large quantity.

Ignitables

Ignitable liquids include both flammables and combustibles. The definitions below are those of the National Fire Protection Association (NFPA) and are used by most fire prevention programs.[3] However, regulatory agencies may use slightly different definitions. For example, the EPA uses the term "ignitable" to refer to liquids with a flash point less than 60 C and to strong oxidizers.[4]

Flammable Liquids

Flammable liquids are those with a very low flash point (the temperature at which a liquid gives off vapors in sufficient concentration to form an ignitable mixture with air), boiling point (at normal atmospheric pressure) or both. Flammable liquids are divided into three groups, with "Class IA" designating the most flammable liquids (Table 3-1). For example, diethyl ether (with a flash point of −45 C) and benzene (with a flash point of −11.1 C) are Class IA liquids. Absolute ethanol has a flash point of 12.8 C and is a Class IB liquid.

Combustible Liquids

Combustible liquids have a flash point that is greater than 37.8 C and are also classified into three groups (Table 3-2). As an example, 37% aqueous formaldehyde (the solution usually referred to

Table 3-1. Flammable Liquids

Class IA: flash point < 22.8 C and boiling point < 37.8 C
Class IB: flash point < 22.8 C and boiling point ≥ 37.8 C
Class IC: flash point ≥ 22.8 C and boiling point < 37.8 C

Table 3-2. Combustible Liquids

Class II: flash point $\geqslant$ 37.8 C and $<$ 60 C
Class IIIA: flash point $\geqslant$ 60 C and $<$ 93.3 C
Class IIIB: flash point $\geqslant$ 93.3 C

as "formalin") has a flash point of 85 C and is therefore in Class IIIA.

Reactive Chemicals

Reactive (explosive) chemicals are those that are capable of violent decomposition at normal temperatures and pressures. For hazardous waste regulations, for example, this term is reserved for chemicals that can undergo violent change normally without detonation or if subjected to a strong initiating source; those that react violently or form a potentially violent mixture in water; or those that are capable of explosive decomposition.[5]

Toxins

Toxin is a term that can refer to almost any substance in quantity. Aspirin, vitamin preparations and other commonly encountered substances have all caused fatal poisonings. Even water can cause an acute intoxication if sufficient quantities are ingested over a short interval. In a safety context, the term is generally applied if a substance that is inhaled, ingested or contacted in small amounts can cause serious biologic effects. The *Registry of Toxic Effects of Chemical Substances*[6] (*RTECS*) subdivides this category.

Irritants

Irritants may be either local or systemic. The term is not usually applied to corrosive substances, however. Irritants may be identified as either "primary skin irritants" or "primary eye irritants" or both, reflecting the test system employed.

Mutagens

Mutagens are chemicals that can cause a hereditable change in genetic material. There are many different mutagenic test systems. Those that involve living species usually measure the effect on lower organisms such as bacteria, fungi or insects. Because of this, the term "mutagen" is frequently applied to substances that have not been shown to cause genetic rearrangements in mammalian species. The *RTECS* has more than 6000 listings of chemicals for which mutagenic data is available.

Reproductive Effects

Reproductive effects are those that affect fertility, cause developmental abnormalities during gestation, or have adverse effects on newborns.

Tumorigens

Tumorigens are substances that have been reported to be associated with benign or malignant tumors. The *RTECS* defines three levels of tumorigenicity.

Carcinogens: Carcinogenic chemicals have been shown to cause malignant neoplasms in animal tests using control animals and valid statistical methods.

Neoplastinogens: Neoplastinogenic chemicals cause tumors that cannot be definitely classified as either benign or malignant. That the data have been derived from controlled experiments and valid statistics is implied in the term.

Equivocal tumorigens: Equivocal tumorigenicity is concluded if the evidence derives from uncontrolled experiments or if the experimental results are otherwise uninterpretable.

The Occupational Safety and Health Administration (OSHA) uses a slightly different definition for the term "carcinogen." Certain compounds such as benzidine and asbestos are specifically regulated because the evidence for carcinogenicity is overwhelming. Currently there are 24 chemicals that are specifically regulated by OSHA.[7] "Potential carcinogens" were also regulated in 1980, but as a conceptual group rather than individually.[8,9] "Category I potential carcinogens" are those that have been shown to cause malignant tumors in humans or in an animal system "in accordance with other scientifically evaluated evidence." The need for extensive medical monitoring and close containment is implied. "Category II potential carcinogens" have been shown to cause malignant tumors in only one animal system but without the same degree of concordance. The chemicals that appear on these two lists are subject to change, and the local office of OSHA should be contacted for the latest information. More recent OSHA publications have cited references from the International Agency for Research on Cancer (IARC), National Toxicology Program (NTP) and American Conference of Governmental Industrial Hygienists (ACGIH) rather than these "potential carcinogen" Department of Labor lists.[10,11]

Exposure Levels and Limits

The mode of contact is an important variable in estimating a substance's toxicity. Short-term exposure produces serious biologic effects in some cases; such chemicals are termed acutely toxic. Standard tests have evolved to measure and define acute toxins. These are usually defined by the dose required to kill 50% of test animals (LD_{50}). The route of administration must be stated. The species of animal in which the substance was tested usually follows the stated dosage. The lower the concentration at which toxic effects can be measured, the more toxic the chemical. For example, "LD_{50}(oral) <50 mg/kg," "LD_{50}(oral) <15 ml/kg" and "LD_{50}(inhalation) <100 ppm" are descriptions of extremely toxic chemicals.

The ACGIH is a widely respected professional organization that makes recommendations on exposure limits based upon the best available information. Sources include industrial experience as well as human and animal studies.[12] Two major types of permissible exposure limits, described as threshold limit values (TLVs), are recognized by the ACGIH. "TLV-TWAs" (TLVs based on 8-hour, time-weighted averages) are used to denote the permissible exposure limits for those substances to which workers are exposed repeatedly, day after day and week after week, without adverse effect. "TLV-STELs" (TLVs based on short-term exposure limits) are the concentrations of vapors to which workers can be exposed continuously for brief periods (15 minutes) without suffering irritation, tissue damage or narcosis. Consulation with a Certified Industrial Hygienist is often very helpful in defining a relevant containment strategy for the chemical vapors resident in a specific work environment.

Radioactive Chemicals

Radioactive chemicals are those that emit ionizing radiation in excess of background levels. In an immunohematology laboratory, radionuclides used in radioligand procedures are likely to be present. The laboratory's Materials License that was issued by the Nuclear Regulatory Commission (NRC) will define the specific radiochemicals and the maximal amounts that may be employed.

Labeling Systems

Room and Cabinet Labels

Room and cabinet labels commonly follow OSHA regulations and NFPA standards. OHSA's General Industry Standards contain an accident-precaution signage system that should be used wherever applicable.[13] Danger signs are indicated in red, black and white; caution signs are indicated in yellow and black; and safety instruction signs are indicated in green and white. This OSHA signage system is direct, but lacks detail. In a laboratory work environment, it can be of significant value to visitors and nontechnical employees.

NFPA 704 specifies the familiar diamond-shaped sign framing the numbers that summarize the fire hazard of the chemicals in a room or of a safety cabinet's contents.[14] Each diamond-shaped sign in this system is divided into four smaller diamonds—a blue diamond on the left containing a number that rates the health hazard of the contents (ie, from fumes evolved during a conflagration); a yellow diamond on the right that rates the chemicals' reactivity (instability); and a red diamond at the pinnacle that rates the materials' flammability. The number within each of these small diamonds will be from 0 (low hazard) to 4 (high hazard). The white diamond in the lowest corner is available for optional, additional symbology. This system is specifically designed for the benefit of firefighters who may be forced to enter the area during a fire. Therefore, its use should be coordinated with the local fire authorities.

Reagent Labels

Reagent labels need different signage. All hazardous chemicals stored or used in amounts that represent a significant danger should carry warning labels. Such labels should be brightly colored and simple enough to import useful information to nonchemists who may be in the vicinity. These labels should comply with the National Committee for Clinical Laboratory Standards'

```
Caution: CORROSIVE
Flush Exposed Area Immediately with Water
Do not store near organic solvents
```

Figure 3-1. Reagent Label.

Standard ASL-1, "Labeling of Laboratory Reagents." Useful examples may be found on some commercial reagent labels (eg, the Saf-T-Data labeling system developed by the JT Baker Chemical Company).[15] The laboratory may choose to develop its own system for uniformity. Figure 3-1 is an example of how the label on concentrated sulfuric acid might read.

Finally, a detailed hazardous chemical labeling system is used by the Department of Transportation (DOT).[16] These DOT placards are designed for use on tank cars, cartage trailers and shipping crates. Smaller versions will be found on the exterior cartons of many bulk reagents. The DOT system is of limited use in the laboratory because it lacks sufficient detail and is rarely used on the primary containment vessel.

Storage

The smaller the quantity of hazardous materials that a laboratory inventories, the better. The chemicals found in laboratories are usually much cheaper than the human resources required to manage them. Laboratory managers who purchase solvents or reagent chemicals in bulk to minimize the unit cost may be committing the laboratory to additional expenses. The shelf lives of chemicals are finite. Partially filled containers of chemicals that have been undisturbed for years are in some laboratory supplies; most such containers will never be reopened but will become part of the laboratory's disposal burden. Storage of bulk chemicals introduces additional, specific hazards. Working quantities of hazardous chemicals should be kept to the smallest amounts possible. A purchasing program that replenishes modest supplies as reagents are consumed will ensure both fresh chemicals and minimal storage problems.

The laboratory's storage system should reflect good safety practices. Solvents and reagents should be stored in an area that is separate from the general workflow. As an example, to store solvents in a chemical fume hood is usually inappropriate because the storage containers will be on a working surface. Cabinetry should be stable and level. Chemical bottle carriers should be used for all vessels larger than 500 ml.

Corrosives

Corrosives must be stored near the floor and ALWAYS below eye level. The storage location must be near running water such as a safety shower and eyewash. Aprons and eye protection must be available (and used!). Signage should be posted that specifies the emergency procedures to be followed in event of accidental spillage, breakage or human exposures. The floor of the storage area should be a basin to trap liquids in the event of breakage or leakage. Oxidizing corrosives (such as concentrated sulfuric or nitric acid) must never be stored near organic solvents or other hydrocarbons.

Ignitables

Ignitable liquids must be stored with special care. Storage should be in accordance with NFPA 30, the Flammable and Combustible Liquids Code.[3] The chosen location must be away from potential sources of ignition and distant from exits and thoroughfares. Safety cans should be used wherever possible. (Safety cans are containers with an automatically closing lid, a flame arrester in the spout and an emergency pressure-release valve.) Flammable-liquid storage cabinets should be provided if moderate amounts of such liquids are to be stocked.[17] The amount that can be stored outside of such a cabinet may not exceed 10 gallons per 5000 square feet. Up to 60 gallons per 5000 square feet may be stored within such cabinets. (Many flammable-liquid storage cabinets are intended for amounts less than 60 gallons; it is important to check the manufacturer's rating for a given cabinet before loading it.)

The typical flammables storage cabinet is sealed (nonvented). Its purpose is to delay the combustion of the contents in the event of surrounding conflagration just long enough to allow personnel egress from the premises. Venting of a cabinet to the outside or into a fume hood exhaust system is permitted, provided that the rating of the ductwork is equal to that of the cabinet.

The size of the individual containers should not exceed the specifications listed in Table 3-3, based upon the ignitability class of the liquid and the container type.[3]

Table 3-3. Container Size for Ignitability

Ignitability Class	Container Type		
	Glass	Metal or Plastic	Safety Can
IA	1 pt	1 gal	2 gal
IB	1 qt	5 gal	5 gal
IC	1 gal	5 gal	5 gal
II	1 gal	5 gal	5 gal
III	5 gal	5 gal	5 gal

Ignitable liquids should not be stored in refrigerators or in environmental cold rooms. If these liquids must be stored in a refrigerator (for example, if the procedure requires cold solvents), the refrigerator should be explosion-proof.

Properly rated fire extinguishing devices must be available wherever flammable and combustible liquids are stored or used.[18] The use of these devices and the proper method for evacuation of the laboratory facility should be part of the training of laboratory employees, especially if the laboratory is located within a hospital.[19]

Carcinogens

Carcinogens and suspect carcinogens should be stored in an area specifically designated. Access to these chemicals must be limited to individuals who understand the hazard and who have been specially trained in safe-handling procedures.

Disposal

The laboratory has a responsibility to the community to ensure that its waste handling policies are carefully defined and properly followed. Some waste can be injurious to those who must handle it; other waste can damage sewage systems and treatment facilities; and many wastes can pollute the environment into which they are discharged or dumped. The responsibility for the containment of these hazards is the waste generator's. This responsibility can neither be assigned nor transferred. The laboratory director or the safety committee must identify those wastes that will require special handling. Some wastes can be discarded into the normal waste stream after treatment to eliminate the hazard (eg, following dilution in waste water effluent, after radioactive decay to de minimis levels or following acid/

base neutralization). Others must be segregated, labeled and shipped elsewhere for disposal.

The Resource Conservation and Recovery Act (RCRA) of 1976 as amended regards hazardous waste as a solid waste, or a combination of solid wastes, which because of its quantity, concentration, physical, chemical or infectious characteristics may either pose a substantial or potential hazard to human health or to the environment.[20] Recent RCRA amendments require generators to certify that they have reduced the volume and toxicity of their hazardous wastes to the "maximum degree economically practicable." Under Congressional charge, the EPA has defined the functional characteristics of hazardous wastes.[21] Laboratory wastes may be considered hazardous because of their flammable, reactive, corrosive, toxic, infectious, phytotoxic, mutagenic, radioactive or carcinogenic characteristics. Proper disposal methods must be specified for each hazardous waste identified. The disposal method of choice will depend upon the type of chemical, the amount, the available facilities and local ordinances.

Radioactive Decay

Radioactive decay on-site should be considered for short half-life radionuclides. The permitted amount will be specified in the institution's Materials License. The goal of this method is to allow the radioactivity of the waste to decrease to the point at which it is indistinguishable from background radiation. A portable survey meter is a convenient device to ascertain this endpoint. (If a portable survey meter is used, however, it must be calibrated with a source traceable to an appropriate National Bureau of Standards referent.) The waste may then be incinerated or mixed with the facility's normal effluent as it enters the sanitary sewage system. NRC tables define the allowable concentrations.[22]

Incineration

Incineration may safely destroy many types of substances. Although incineration is most applicable to the disposal of biohazardous wastes, ignitable solvents may be injected into an appropriate combustion chamber to render them harmless to the environment. This requires an incinerator of special design and a specific permit from the EPA. Trial burns are a prerequisite to demonstrate the destruction efficiency. Incineration should be seriously considered for destruction of highly toxic and environmentally persistent chemicals.

Recycling

Recycling possibilities should be investigated for selected chemicals. Metallic mercury, silver salts and organic solvents are among the chemicals most often reclaimed, distilled, purified and reused. Although recycling methods may achieve an environmental ideal, they can be expensive. Distillation of flammable liquids can be extremely hazardous. Laboratories that have chosen distillation and reclamation as waste disposal methods usually have the process performed by outside specialists.

Chemical exchanges should also be investigated by laboratorians interested in recycling. Informal exchanges may be found in classified advertisements in trade publications, and some large campuses have organized their own programs. Brokerages exist to bring together those with surplus or waste chemicals and potential users of these materials.

Disposal at a Remote Facility

The best disposal methods are those that eliminate the hazard at the generator's facility. Less desired, but often the only alternative, is disposal at a remote facility. Such facilities include recycling centers, licensed incinerators and sanitary landfills. Selection of a disposal facility, no matter how appropriate to the chemical waste, does not transfer the environmental responsibility from the generator to the disposal or storage agent. The environmental responsibility remains with the generating facility even after many years of storage. All hazardous wastes shipped off-site should have a detailed shipping manifest that identifies the type and quantity of the wastes being transported. These records must be kept for 3 years,[23] and probably should be maintained as long as the material may continue to be hazardous to the environment.

"Small containers of hazardous waste in over-packed drums" are referred to colloquially as "lab packs."[24] These are 55-gallon steel drums filled with smaller, individual containers that in turn are surrounded by absorbing material such as vermiculite or fuller's earth. Incompatible chemicals may not be stored in the same drum, and complete manifesting is required.

Evaporation

Evaporation may be appropriate for disposal of small quantities of ignitable solvents. The method chosen must not violate EPA standards or good fire prevention practices. Small amounts of diethyl ether, for example, may be evaporated in a properly vented chemical fume hood that has a face velocity of at least 100 feet per minute or may be poured outdoors into a slag, evaporation pit that is located well away from inhabited buildings.

Chemical Decomposition and Degradation

Chemical decomposition and degradation may be employed for selected chemicals. Waste acids may be neutralized in limestone tanks. The flushing effluent from these tanks may safely enter the sanitary sewer with permission of the local sewer authorities. Many other hazardous reagent chemicals can also be rendered nonhazardous after treatment at the generator's facility. Appropriate design of such treatment systems demands considerable knowledge of the chemistry involved, and should only be planned after consultation with experts.[25]

Documentation of Safe Work Practices

The manager of a clinical laboratory should consider documenting safe work practices in the same manner as analytic quality is documented.[26] This facilitates supervisory review of compliance with the procedures specified in the manuals and required for accreditation. To document these practices also provides continuous reinforcement for those technologists who are at primary risk. Moreover, supervisory review of the documentation assures the technical staff that management is sincerely concerned with their health and welfare.

Certain documents are required by regulatory agencies. The EPA demands that generators of hazardous waste keep records of the amounts generated and the disposition of these chemicals. These regulations pertain to any business that generates more than 100 kg hazardous waste per month,[27] which includes nearly all hospitals. The Occupational Safety and Health Administration requires documentation of serious accidents (see below). The use of radionuclides is regulated by the Nuclear Regulatory Commission.[28] Shipment of hazardous materials is regulated by the Department of Transportation.[29] For those laboratories engaged in interstate commerce and/or who are seeking Medicare reimbursement, the Clinical Laboratory Improvement Act of 1967 and amendments to the Medicare Act have authorized the Health Care Financing Administration to enforce compliance with regulations that address safe work practices. State licensure policies and local ordinances may impose additional documentary requirements.

Many clinical laboratories participate voluntarily in the accreditation programs of the American Association of Blood Banks and of the College of American Pathologists. Hospital laboratories may also be inspected by the Joint Commission on Accreditation of Hospitals. Assurance of hazard containment within the facility and promotion of safe work practices are essential for accreditation by these programs. Appropriate definition of safe work practices and careful documentation of compliance with the defined standards will reassure the inspectors from regulatory and accrediting agencies that the laboratory has a well-managed safety program.

The documentation of a chemical safety program should begin with the safety manual. There are many useful references and models that can be adapted to a laboratory's needs.[30-33] Under no circumstances, however, should a manual that was originally written for another laboratory be adopted without careful review. The production of a safety manual is the unassignable responsibility of the laboratory director. The authorship of the safety manual may be delegated, but the responsibility for its contents may never be avoided.

If the laboratory already has a safety manual, the director must be prepared to demonstrate that it has been reviewed regularly for accuracy and completeness. This is often delegated to a safety committee, the members of which have a thorough knowledge of hazard containment practices and an active interest in laboratory safety. The safety committee may be charged with orientation of new employees and with the continuing education in safe work practices of experienced laboratorians. Employees who demonstrate familiarity with the safety manual's contents should receive regular, positive reinforcement. Supervisors should document this familiarity and incorporate the record into the employees' personnel files.

The safety manual should not be the laboratory's only code of safe working procedures. Each analytic procedure that has inherent chemical hazards should itemize the safety equipment needed among its list of specified materials. This may include personal, protective equipment such as pipetting aids, gloves, respirators and aprons; or it may specify that a chemical fume hood be employed. The appropriate route for discarding waste chemicals and soiled disposables should be clearly evident from the text of the procedure. The annual review of such procedures is an opportune time for the director to determine whether the safe work practices that are appropriate for each laboratory process are explicit within the text of the procedure. It may also be appropriate to document compliance with these procedures. The rigor with which these safe work practices must be recorded depends upon the types of hazards being contained and the customs of the laboratory. Histopathology laboratory directors, for example, may elect to monitor ambient levels of potentially toxic fumes and to record the readings.

Even in the safest laboratories, accidents will occur. Reporting of occupational injuries and illnesses is required by the Occupational Safety and Health Act of 1970. Occupational injuries include cuts, fractures, sprains, burns, etc, that have followed a work accident or that derive from a single-incident exposure in the work environment. An occupational illness can be any abnormal condition or disorder (other than one resulting from an occupational injury) caused by exposure to employment-related, environmental factors. This includes the effects of chronic exposure to toxic chemicals. Any fatality, injury resulting in the hospitalization of three or more employees, property damage exceeding $25,000, biologic exposure resulting in lost time or involving the public and accidents resulting in spillage of radioactive materials are defined as "serious accidents" and are reportable to OSHA. Each illness or nonfatal injury that requires transfer to another job, termination or treatment (other than first aid) must be logged within 6 working days of discovery.[34] Hospital risk managers will usually require that minor accidents such as falls, spills and needlesticks be recorded for liability considerations.

Each such accident or incident should be investigated. The safety committee or the laboratory director should always review the safety manual and the procedures manual to determine whether standard operating practices were being followed at the time. An update of these manuals must be considered if all personnel were discharging their duties as directed at the time. More commonly, however, the incident would have been avoided if procedures had been followed as defined. Such a conclusion should set specific goals for the continuing education program. No form of reinforcement of the importance of safe work practices will be more effective than the bad example set by the injury of a coworker.

A Chemical Hygiene Plan

OSHA has published its intention to require all laboratories that use hazardous chemicals—clinical, academic and industrial—to develop a chemical hygiene plan (CHP).[10] If promulgated, the Department of Labor will mandate that all laboratory employers develop a written, comprehensive plan that addresses each hazardous chemical stored and used on the premises. Whether or not a written CHP will be required by OSHA, this proposal is a useful focus for discussing a substance-specific, chemical safety program.

Development of a CHP begins with a thorough chemical inventory. The safety director or the safety committee must determine the location and the amount of each hazardous chemical employed in the laboratory. This can be a laborious task. Most substances encountered will be in small quantity. Some will be aqueous dilutions. Vessels labeled by their manufacturers may have only proprietary information that lack chemical formulae; such substances should be noted as needing special review. The more comprehensive the inventory, however, the less likely will be inadvertent, but significant, omissions.

The second step is to gather the needed toxicity data for each identified chemical. The primary source of information for each substance should be its vendor. OSHA requires each distributor of a hazardous material to provide a Material Safety Data Sheet (MSDS) upon request. The request for a MSDS should be included within the purchase order for each hazardous material. The format of a MSDS is standardized and includes information on toxicity, routine handling precautions, emergency procedures in the event of accidential exposure and recommendations for spill cleanup. To have the relevant MSDSs at hand is not only useful, it may be required by local ordinance. Many communities have "right to know" laws which ensure that employees who must handle or work in the vicinity of hazardous chemicals have access to such information. The typical MSDS is directed to industrial-scale uses of the chemical in question; the chemical safety committee may need to annotate the text to make it applicable to laboratory-scale quantities.

It is not always possible to acquire a MSDS for a hazardous chemical identified during the inventory process that was purchased in years past. The safety director may judge that some of the MSDSs provided are lacking in sufficient detail to be useful in a laboratory application. Furthermore, reagent chemicals for which the toxic potential is unclear must be researched, and new scientific evidence for toxicity may be pertinent. For these reasons, additional sources of information may need to be consulted.

The *Registry of Toxic Effects of Chemical Substances* (*RTECS*) is published by the National Institutes of Occupational Safety and Health (NIOSH) of the Department of Health and Human Services. It contains over 65,000 entries cross-indexed under a quarter-million chemical names. This registry, which is continuously updated, is available in print both in book format and in a quarterly microfiche edition. It may also be accessed through the National Library of Medicine Medical Literature Analysis and Retrieval System (MEDLARS) and the National Institutes of Health/Environmental Protection Agency Chemical Information System (CIS).

There are several abstract services that can be consulted for useful chemical information. Chemical Abstracts Service (CAS) is probably the most familiar, with over two million citations. It is also available on-line. *Chemical Abstracts* is produced by Chemical Abstracts Service, P.O. Box 3012, Columbus, Ohio, 43210.

Laboratorians concerned about carcinogens and substances that are considered to be potentially carcinogenic should be aware of the IARC and the NTP. The International Agency for Research on Cancer (IARC) is an agency of the World Health Organization. Since 1972 the IARC has published over 30 monographs evaluating the carcinogenic risk of chemicals to man. The National Toxicology Program (NTP) of the US Public Health Service issues a periodic *Annual Report on Carcinogens*. The most recent report was published in 1985.[35] Each report itemizes those substances that are either "known to be carcinogens" or are "reasonably anticipated to be carcinogens." The scope of the NTP is limited to those substances "to which a significant number of persons residing in the United States are exposed."[36]

The National Fire Protection Association is an organization that publishes the National Fire Code, a series of voluntary standards that are written by technical experts selected from a variety of disciplines. Codes such as NFPA 101 (the "Life Safety Code") and NFPA 70 (the "National Electrical Code") are the bases for many local fire ordinances. Laboratorians should certainly be aware of NFPA 99, which is the "Standard for Health Care Facilities." Workers in research laboratories may need to refer to NFPA 45, the "Standard on Fire Protection for Laboratories Using Chemicals." Both NFPA 99 and NFPA 45 cross-reference to NFPA 30, the "Flammable and Combustible Liquids Code." NFPA 325M, "Fire Hazard Properties of Flammable Liquids, Gases and Volatile Solids," is a compendium of information about the ignitability and reactivity of many commonly encountered chemicals. It is the best source for defining the signage and specifying the limitations on the contents of flammables storage cabinetry.

An ongoing hazardous chemical information program may be an appropriate part of the laboratory's reagent chemical inventory management system. Such a program can also provide an internal mechanism for assessing the completeness of the laboratory's hazardous chemical waste accounting.

Chemicals of Interest to Blood Banking Specialists

The following are recommendations that have been abstracted from several sources, including the HAZARDLINE Database™ (BRS/Saunders, New York, NY) and the *Registry of Toxic Effects of Chemical Substances* (*RTECS*) from the National Institute for Occupational Safety and Health (NIOSH). The original sources should be consulted for updates. Reference material safety data sheets and ACGIH tables were also used.[37,38]

The Comprehensive Environmental Response, Compensation and Liability Act (CERCLA) of 1980 defines the liability of a generator of hazardous waste for damage to the environment under the Federal Water Control Act, Section 311(b)(2)(A); the Solid Waste Disposal Act, Section 3001; the Clean Water Act, Section 307(A); the Clean Air Act, Section 112; the Toxic Substances Control Act, Section 7; and under CERCLA, Section 102. The CERCLA hazard ratings listed in the following discussions, therefore, are a measure of risk following spills or improper waste disposal. The CERCLA hazard rating system consists of four categories. Each category is graded on a scale from 0 (minimally hazardous) to 4 (extremely hazardous). The first three categories (health hazard, ignitability and reactivity) are essentially identical to those used in the rating system used by the NFPA.[14] The fourth (persistence or biodegradability) is defined in EPA regulations.[39]

Chloroform

Chloroform (Table 3-4) is a colorless, heavy, volatile liquid that has a sweetish taste. It is nonflammable and noncombustible. (However, in a fire, chloroform may evolve phosgene gas, which is extremely toxic.) The boiling point is 62 C. Permissible exposure levels are 10 ppm TWA (ACGIH), 50 ppm ceiling

(OSHA-adopted for effects other than cancer) and 2 ppm 60-min ceiling (NIOSH). Chloroform is a "suspect human carcinogen" as defined by the IARC, NTP and ACGIH. NIOSH also recommends that this substance be treated as a potential carcinogen.[40] It is an animal carcinogen (IARC). Teratogenic and mutagenic data have been published.

Chloroform is a primary skin irritant, a central nervous system depressant, a nephrotoxin and a hepatotoxin. Acute exposure to chloroform causes excitation, dizziness, nausea and headache, followed by unconsciousness and respiratory failure. Death may occur from cardiac arrest or from hepatic damage. Chronic inhalation may result in liver or kidney damage. The odor threshold is 100 ppm, but chloroform has poor warning properties since olfactory fatigue occurs. Exposure may be by inhalation, ingestion or skin or eye contact. If the material gets into the eyes, immediately wash the eyes with large amounts of water and seek medical attention immediately. If chloroform gets on the skin, wash with soap or mild detergent and water. In inhalation overexposure, remove the victim from the area to fresh air, maintain an airway and respiration and seek medical attention immediately. After accidental ingestion, have a victim who is conscious drink large amounts of water and induce vomiting. Do not make an unconscious or stuporous victim vomit. Get medical attention immediately. Table 3-5 summarizes the toxicity levels that have been cited by NIOSH.[6]

Safety goggles should be worn when working with this substance. Contact lenses should not be worn when working with this material. Clothing that becomes soaked with this chemical must be removed immediately and placed in a closed container until it can be discarded or cleaned; the person performing the cleaning should be informed of the nature of the contaminant. Waste disposal is regulated under the RCRA. The EPA number for chloroform is U044. CERCLA hazard ratings: toxicity = 3; ignitability = 0; reactivity = 0; persistence = 3.

Table 3-4. Chloroform

Synonyms: Trichloromethane. Methane trichloride. Methenyl trichloride. NCI-CO2686. Cobehn Spray-clean solvent. Formyl trichloride. Freon 20. Trichloroform. Refrigerant R 20. CAS #000-067-663.

Chemical formula: $CHCl_3$

MW: 119.4 daltons

Table 3-5. Toxicity Levels of Chloroform

ORL-HMN LD$_{Lo}$	=	140 mg/kg
IHL-RAT LC$_{Lo}$	=	8000 ppm/4 hr
IHL-HMN TC$_{Lo}$	=	1000 mg/m^3/1 hr
IHL-MUS LC$_{50}$	=	28 g/m^3
IHL-HMN TC$_{Lo}$	=	5000 mg/m^3/7 min
IHL-DOG LC$_{50}$	=	100 g/m^3
UNK-MAN LD$_{Lo}$	=	546 mg/kg
IHL-CAT LC$_{LO}$	=	35,000 mg/m^3/4 hr
ORL-RAT LD$_{50}$	=	1194 mg/kg
IHL-RBT LC$_{50}$	=	59 g/m^3
ORL-MUS LD$_{50}$	=	80 mg/kg
IHL-GPG LC$_{Lo}$	=	20,000 ppm/2 hr
ORL-DOG LD$_{Lo}$	=	1000 mg/kg
IHL-MAM LC$_{Lo}$	=	25,000 ppm/5 min
ORL-RBT LD$_{Lo}$	=	500 mg/kg

Route of administration:

ORL	=	oral
IHL	=	inhalation
UNK	=	unreported

Animal species tested:

DOG	=	dog
CAT	=	cat
GPG	=	guinea pig
HMN	=	human
MAM	=	mammal (species unspecified)
MAN	=	man
RAT	=	rat
MUS	=	mouse
RBT	=	rabbit

Measurement:

LC$_{50}$	=	concentration required to kill 50% of test animals
LD$_{50}$	=	lethal dose for 50% of test animals
LC$_{Lo}$	=	lowest published lethal concentration
LD$_{Lo}$	=	lowest published lethal dose
TC$_{Lo}$	=	lowest published toxic concentration

Copper Sulfate

Copper sulfate (Table 3-6) occurs naturally as light blue or grayish-white to greenish-white crystals and as amorphous powder. It is hygroscopic, soluble in water and nonflammable. *RTECS* rates it as an indefinite carcinogen. Mutagenic data are available (*RTECS*). ACGIH has set no permissible exposure limits. Copper sulfate is an irritant that can be poisonous if ingested, inhaled or after contact with skin or eyes. Symptoms

Table 3-6. Copper Sulfate

Synonyms: Cupric sulfate. Copper (II) sulfate. Blue copper. Blue stone. Blue vitriol. Griffin Super Cu. CAS #007-758-987.

Chemical formula: $CuSO_4$ or $CuSO_4 \cdot 5H_2O$

MW: 159.6 (anhydrous) or 249.7 (hydrated) daltons

Table 3-7. Toxicity Levels of Copper Sulfate

ORL-CHD TD_{Lo}	= 200 mg/kg
ORL-HMN TD_{Lo}	= 50 mg/kg
ORL-HMN TD_{Lo}	= 11 mg/kg

Route of administration:
ORL   = oral
Animal species tested:
CHD   = child
HMN   = human
Measurement:
TD_{Lo} = lowest published toxic dose

include inflammation, headache, metallic taste in the mouth, salivation, sweating, methemoglobinemia, nausea, vomiting, diarrhea and in extreme exposures gastrointestinal bleeding, oliguria, hypotension and hemolytic anemia. Toxicity levels are shown in Table 3-7.

Copper sulfate should not be stored near hydroxylamine, magnesium, aluminum power, acetylene gas or sodium hypobromite. Thermal decomposition products can be toxic. Skin or clothing that becomes contaminated with copper salts should be washed with mild detergent and copious amounts of water. Emergency treatment of ingestion should include dilution with water or milk, induction of vomiting (if the patient is conscious) and prompt medical attention. CERCLA hazard ratings: toxicity = 3; ignitability = 0; reactivity = 0; persistence = 3.

Ethyl Ether

Ethyl ether (Table 3-8) is a colorless, volatile, hygroscopic liquid that has an aromatic odor and a burning, sweet taste. Ether is moderately soluble in water. The flash point is -45 C and the boiling point is 34 C (NFPA Class I flammable liquid). Permissible exposures are 400 ppm TWA (OSHA, ACGIH) and 500 ppm STEL (ACGIH), set to prevent irritation and central nervous system depression. The odor threshold (1.0 ppm) is well below the permissible exposure level.

Ethyl ether is a mild eye and mucous membrane irritant, a primary skin irritant and a central nervous system depressant. Acute exposure can cause anesthetic effects, such as vomiting and excitement, that lead to unconsciousness, coma and respiratory paralysis. Nasal irritation provides adequate warning properties well below the anesthetic-effects concentration. Exposure may be by inhalation, ingestion or skin or eye contact. If ether accidentally splashes into the eyes, immediately wash the victim's eyes with large amounts of water and seek medical attention immediately. If this chemical contacts the skin, wash with soap or mild detergent and water. Clothing that has been soaked in ether must be removed immediately and discarded outdoors or dried in a chemical fume hood. In inhalation overexposure, remove the victim from the area to fresh air; maintain airway and respiration and get medical attention immediately. After accidental ingestion, have a conscious victim drink large amounts of water and induce vomiting. Do not make an unconscious or stuporous victim vomit. Seek medical attention immediately. Toxicity data are shown in Table 3-9. OSHA and NIOSH have set the "dangerous exposure concentration" at 19,000 ppm.

Ethyl ether should be stored away from strong oxidizers such as sulfuric acid, nitric acid, oxygen and peroxides. Protect from light. Explosive peroxides can form during storage. The risk of peroxide formation is increased after opening a container of anhydrous ether and exposing the contents to air. The peroxides formed can combine with the walls of the vessel, rendering the vessel potentially explosive even after it is empty. Glass is at high risk for peroxide formation; therefore, ethyl ether should

Table 3-8. Ethyl Ether

Synonyms: Diethyl ether. Ethyl oxide. Diethyl oxide. Solvent ether. Ethoxyethane. 1,1-oxybisethane. Anesthetic ether. 3-oxapentane. Fulfuric ether. Pronarcol. CAS #000-060-297.

Chemical formula: $C_2H_5OC_2H_5$

MW: 74.1 daltons

never be stored in glass. Lead-lined containers decrease the risk, as does the addition of water. Ethyl ether should always be purchased in the smallest containers feasible and then stored in the original vessels. Ether must be stored in a well-ventilated area. Refrigerators—even explosion-proof refrigerators—are not recommended. Storage in a flammables storage cabinet is acceptable, but this material is so volatile that the cabinet should be vented to the outdoors. Vapors that accumulate in an enclosed space (such as a cabinet) can explode when the cabinet is opened, even though the point of ignition may be many feet away.

Protective clothing and eye protection should be worn when pouring or mixing this substance. Gloves made of polyurethane, polyvinyl alcohol, butyl rubber, neoprene/styrene-butadiene rubber, nitrile rubber, polyethylene and chlorinated polyethylene are acceptable. Contact lenses should not be worn without eye protection when working with this chemical.

Ethyl ether is regulated as a hazardous waste under the RCRA. The EPA hazardous waste number for ethyl ether is

Table 3-9. Toxicity Levels of Ethyl Ether

ORL-MAN LD_{Lo}	= 260 mg/kg
ORL-HMN LD_{Lo}	= 420 mg/kg
IHL-HMN TC_{Lo}	= 200 ppm
ORL-RAT LD_{50}	= 1215 mg/kg
IHL-RAT LC_{50}	= 73,000 ppm/150 min
IHL-MUS LC_{50}	= 65,000 ppm/100 min
IHL-DOG LC_{Lo}	= 76,000 ppm
IHL-RBT LC_{Lo}	= 106,000 ppm

Route of administration:
ORL	= oral
IHL	= inhalation

Animal species tested:
DOG	= dog
HMN	= human
MAN	= man
RAT	= rat
MUS	= mouse
RBT	= rabbit

Measurement:
LC_{50}	= concentration required to kill 50% of test animals
LD_{50}	= lethal dose for 50% of test animals
LC_{Lo}	= lowest published lethal concentration
LD_{Lo}	= lowest published lethal dose
TC_{Lo}	= lowest published toxic concentration

U117. CERCLA hazard ratings: toxicity = 2; ignitability = 3; reactivity = 1; persistence = 0. CO_2 and dry chemical fire extinguishers are appropriate for quenching small fires; polymer foam should be used for larger fires.

Glutaraldehyde

Glutaraldehyde (Table 3-10) is colorless and soluble in water. It is rated by the NTP as an experimental carcinogen. Data on mutagenic and reproductive effects are available (*RTECS*). Permissible exposure (ceiling) = 0.2 ppm (ACGIH), set at a level to prevent irritation. It is primarily an irritant of the eyes, skin and respiratory system, but in high concentrations can affect the nervous system. Symptoms of poisoning from inhalation, skin absorption or ingestion include coughing, dyspnea, dizziness, drowsiness, constipation and nausea. Vapors may be very irritating, and therefore provide an element of warning; the odor threshold = 0.3 ppm in air. Toxicity levels are listed in Table 3-11.

Gloves made of butyl rubber, polyurethane, polyethylene, polyvinyl chloride, styrene-butadiene, polyvinyl alcohol or Viton should be worn when working with this agent. Skin or clothing that becomes contaminated should be washed immediately and thoroughly. Contact lenses should not be worn without eye protection when working with this chemical. If glutaraldehyde gets in the eyes, wash the victim's eyes immediately with copious amounts of water and seek medical attention. After accidental ingestion, conscious victims should be encouraged to drink large amounts of water or milk and to vomit. Do not give sodium bicarbonate because this potentiates the toxicity.

Glutaraldehyde is nonflammable, but when heated it may decompose and emit acrid smoke and fumes. Fires in the vicinity should be controlled with carbon dioxide, dry chemical, foam or water fog. CERCLA hazard ratings: toxicity = 2; ignitability = 0; reactivity = 0; persistence = 0.

Table 3-10. Gluteraldehyde

Synonyms: Cidex. 1,5-pentanedione. 1,5-pentanedial. Glutaric dialdehyde. NCI-C22425. Sonacide. Glutaral. CAS #000-111-308.

Chemical formula: OHC_3H_6CHO

MW: 100.1 daltons

Table 3-11. Toxicity Levels of Gluteraldehyde

ORL-RAT LD_{50}	$= 239$ mg/kg
ORL-MUS LD_{50}	$= 231$ mg/kg
IHL-RAT LC_{Lo}	$= 5000$ ppm/4 hr
SKN-RBT LD_{50}	$= 2560$ mg/kg
IPR-MUS LD_{50}	$= 13,900$ μg/kg
IPR-RAT LD_{50}	$= 17,900$ μg/kg

Route of administration:
      ORL   = oral
      IHL   = inhalation
      SKN   = administration onto skin
      IPR   = intraperitoneal injection
Animal species tested:
      RAT   = rat
      MUS = mouse
      RBT   = rabbit
Measurement:
      LD_{50} = lethal dose for 50% of test animals
      LC_{Lo} = lowest published lethal concentration

Phenol

Phenol (Table 3-12) is a colorless or pinkish, hygroscopic, crystalline solid that has a sharp, sweet, tarry odor. It is often used in disinfectant solutions. Permissible exposure limits: 5 ppm (or 19 mg/m^3) TWA (OSHA, NIOSH, ACGIH-skin); 10 ppm (or 38 mg/m^3) STEL (ACGIH-skin). The odor threshold (0.05 ppm) is considered an adequate warning. Phenol is a mucous membrane and skin irritant and a convulsant neurotoxin. Toxicity levels are listed in Table 3-13.

A concentration of 100 ppm is considered immediately dangerous to life and health. Mutagenic data, reproductive data and tumorigenic data are available in the *RTECS*. Phenol is rapidly absorbed through the skin. Symptoms include sweating, thirst, nausea, vomiting, diarrhea, stupor and shock. Eye injuries are especially dangerous; phenol may cause severe ocular damage and blindness. Flush eyes with copious amounts of water and seek immediate medical attention. Remove contaminated clothing from a victim and wash skin with copious amounts of water and a mild detergent. Safety goggles, gloves and aprons must be worn when working with this chemical.

Do not store phenol with peroxides, acetaldehyde, aluminum trichloride or calcium hypochlorite. Contact with strong oxidizers may cause fires and explosions. Contact with reducing

Table 3-12. Phenol

Synonyms: Carbolic acid. Hydroxybenzene. Phenic acid. Phenylic acid. Mono-hydroxybenzene. CAS #000-108-952.

Chemical formula: C_6H_5OH

MW: 94 daltons

Table 3-13. Toxicity Levels of Phenol

ORL-MAN LD_{Lo}	= 140 mg/kg
ORL-RAT LD_{50}	= 414 mg/kg
IHL-RAT LC_{50}	= 316 mg/m^3
SKN-RAT LD_{50}	= 669 mg/kg

Route of administration:		
	ORL	= oral
	IHL	= inhalation
	SKN	= administration onto skin
Animal species tested:		
	MAN	= man
	RAT	= rat
Measurement:		
	LC_{50}	= concentration required to kill 50% of test animals
	LD_{50}	= lethal dose for 50% of test animals
	LD_{Lo}	= lowest published lethal dose

agents may generate H_2 gas. The CERCLA hazard rating is health = 3; ignitability = 2; reactivity = 0; persistence = 1. The NFPA hazard rating is health = 3; ignitability = 2; reactivity = 0. The flash point = 79 C, and the boiling point = 182 C. The RCRA number of phenol is U188. CO_2, dry chemical, foam or water fog extinguishers should be used on small fires involving this agent.

Sodium Hypochlorite Aqueous Solution (5-12%)

Sodium hypochlorite solution (Table 3-14) is a clear, pale yellow or greenish liquid with a chlorine odor. No TLV has been established. The ORL-RAT $LD_{50} \cong 12$ mg/kg for a 12% solution; a 5% solution is reported to be much less toxic. The pH is 9 to 10,

Table 3-14. Sodium Hypochlorite Aqueous Solution (5-12%)

Synonyms: Soda bleach liquor. Antiformin. Household bleach. Chlorox. Purex. Sunny Sol bleach. CAS #007-681-529.

Solute formula: NaClHO

Solute MW: 75.4 daltons

depending upon the sodium hydroxide content. Chlorine is liberated on contact with acid; therefore, it should not be stored with acids. Other incompatibilities include ammonia, urea, oxidizable materials and metals such as Ni, Cu, Sn, Mn and Fe.

Toxicity is due to alkalinity, Cl_2 generation and oxidant properties. Ingestion of a few ounces of a 12% solution can cause corrosion of mucous membranes and perforation of the esophagus or stomach. Contact lenses should not be worn without eye protection when pouring or mixing this chemical. If accidental eye exposure occurs, immediately wash the eyes with large amounts of water and get medical attention immediately. Accidental skin or clothing contamination should be treated with mild detergent and copious amounts of water. Mix and use only in areas with adequate ventilation.

Xylene

Xylene (Table 3-15) is a colorless, aromatic liquid that is essentially insoluble in water (0.00003%). "Xylene" is typically a mixture of ortho-, meta- and paraxylene. The flash point is 29-32 C and the boiling point is 14 C (NFPA combustible liquid Class II). (Note, however, that impurities may lower the flash point to as low as 17 C, such that the ignitability of waste xylene may be greater than that of the analytic grade.) Permissible exposure limits are 100 ppm 8-hr TWA (OSHA, NIOSH and ACGIH), 150 ppm STEL (ACGIH), and 200 ppm 10-minute ceiling (NIOSH). The odor threshold (0.5 ppm) is far smaller than the permissible exposure levels. Teratogenic and mutagenic data are available (*RTECS*). Xylene is listed as an experimental carcinogen by the NTP. Toxicity levels are listed in Table 3-16.

Xylene is a mild eye and mucous membrane irritant and a central nervous system depressant. Ingestion causes severe gastrointestinal upset and may lead to aspiration. Direct eye exposure can cause conjunctivitis and corneal burns. Irritant

Table 3-15. Xylene

Synonyms: Xylol. Dimethylbenzene. Violet 3. Dilan. NCI-C55232.

Chemical formula: $C_6H_4(CH_3)_2$

MW: 106 daltons

Table 3-16. Toxicity Levels of Xylene

IHL-HMN TC_{Lo}	= 200 ppm
IHL-MAN LC_{Lo}	= 10,000 ppm/6 hr
IHL-RAT LC_{50}	= 5000 ppm/4 hr
ORL-RAT LD_{50}	= 4300 mg/kg

Route of administration:
ORL	= oral
IHL	= inhalation

Animal species tested:
HMN	= human
MAN	= man
RAT	= rat

Measurement:
LC_{50}	= concentration required to kill 50% of test animals
LD_{50}	= lethal dose for 50% of test animals
LC_{Lo}	= lowest published lethal concentration
TC_{Lo}	= lowest published toxic concentration

effects and a low odor threshold provide adequate warning properties. Contact lenses should not be worn without eye protection when pouring or mixing this chemical. If accidental eye exposure occurs, immediately wash the eyes with large amounts of water and get medical attention immediately. Accidental skin or clothing contamination should be treated with mild detergent and copious amounts of water. If a victim breaths large amounts of the vapors, move the exposed person to fresh air at once; if breathing has stopped, perform artificial respiration. Get medical attention as soon as possible. If the chemical has been accidentally swallowed, do *not* induce vomiting; get medical attention immediately and remove by gastric lavage and catharsis.

This substance is listed as a hazardous waste by EPA under the RCRA as U239. Xylene should not be stored with strong oxidizers such as sulfuric acid, nitric acid, heat, oxygen or peroxides. Bind and ground metal containers when transferring this liquid. Xylene is explosive at high temperatures. Thermal decomposition products are hazardous and/or toxic. Small fires should be quenched with dry chemical, foam, CO_2, water fog or steam; do not spray with water-stream extinguisher devices. CERCLA hazard ratings: toxicity = 2; ignitability = 3; reactivity = 0; persistence = 1.

References

1. National Association of Corrosion Engineers. Standard TM-01-69: Test methods for the evaluation of solid waste, physical/chemical methods.
2. Title 40, Code of Federal Regulations, Part 261, Subpart C, §261.22.
3. National Fire Protection Association. NFPA 30-1984: Flammable and Combustible Liquids Code.
4. Title 40, Code of Federal Regulations, Part 261, Subpart C, §261.21.
5. Title 40, Code of Federal Regulations, Part 261, Subpart C, §261.23.
6. National Institute of Occupational Safety and Health. Registry of toxic effects of chemical substances.
7. Title 29, Code of Federal Regulations Part 1910, Subpart Z, §1910.1001-1047.
8. Title 29, Code of Federal Regulations Part 1990, §1990.112.
9. Federal Register 45(157):53672-53679 (August 12, 1980).
10. Federal Register 51(142):26660-26684 (July 24, 1986).
11. Occupational Safety and Health Administration. OSHA industrial hygiene technical manual. US Department of Labor, 1984.
12. American Conference of Governmental and Industrial Hygienists. TLVs. Threshold limit values for chemical substances in the work environment adopted by ACGIH with intended changes for 1985-86. Cincinnati: ACGIH, 1985.
13. Title 29, Code of Federal Regulations, Part 1910, Subpart J, §1910.145.
14. National Fire Protection Association. NFPA 704-1980: Standard system for the identification of the fire hazards of materials.
15. Pipitone DA, ed. Safe storage of laboratory chemicals. New York: John Wiley and Sons, 1984.
16. Title 49, Code of Federal Regulations, Parts 100-177 (especially Part 172, Subpart E, §172.400-406).
17. National Fire Protection Association. NFPA 99-1987: Health care facilities, Chapter 10, §10-7.
18. National Fire Protection Association. NFPA 10: Portable fire extinguishers.

19. National Fire Protection Association. NFPA 101: Life safety code.
20. 42 USC §6901 et seq.
21. Title 40, Code of Federal Regulations, Parts 260-264.
22. Title 10, Code of Federal Regulations, Part 20, Appendix B, Table II.
23. Title 40, Code of Federal Regulations, Part 263, Subpart B, §263.20-263.22.
24. Title 40, Code of Federal Regulations, Part 264, Subpart N, §264.316.
25. National Research Council (US). Committee on Hazardous Substances in the Laboratory. Prudent practices for disposal of chemicals from laboratories. Washington, DC: National Academy Press, 1983.
26. Hoeltge GA. Documentation of safe work practices in the clinical laboratory. Clin Lab Med (in press).
27. Title 40, Code of Federal Regulations, Part 262, Subpart D, §262.44.
28. Title 10, Code of Federal Regulations, Chapter I (especially Parts 30-35, 40, 70).
29. Title 49, Code of Federal Regulations, Subchapter C, Parts 171-179.
30. Manufacturing Chemists Association. Guide for safety in the chemical laboratory. New York: Van Nostrand Reinhold Company, 1972.
31. Flury PA, DeLuca K. Environmental health and safety in the hospital laboratory. Springfield, Illinois: Charles C Thomas, 1978.
32. Hawk WA, Hoeltge G, Sodeman TM. Guidelines for laboratory safety in the clinical laboratory. College of American Pathologists, 1984.
33. Miller BM et al, eds. Laboratory safety: principles and practices. Washington, DC: American Society for Microbiology, 1986.
34. Title 29, Code of Federal Regulations, Part 1904.2.
35. US Department of Health and Human Services. Fourth annual report on carcinogens: Summary 1985. NTP 85-002.
36. Public Law 95-622, §262, Paragraph (4).
37. Nielson JM, ed. Material safety data sheets collection. Schenectady, NY: General Electric Co, 1980.
38. American Conference of Government Industrial Hygienists. TLVs: Threshold limit values and biological exposure indices for 1985-86. 2nd printing. Cincinnati: ACGIH, 1986.
39. Title 40, Code of Federal Regulations, Part 300, Appendix A, para. 3.4.
40. Anonymous. NIOSH recommendations, for occupational safety and health standards. MMWR (suppl) 1986; 35:1s-35s.

In: Gibbs, FL and Kasprisin, CA, eds.
Environmental Safety in the Blood Bank
Arlington, VA: American Association
of Blood Banks, 1987

4

Handling Infectious Agents in the Blood Bank

Serl E. Rosenschein, MD

*T*HE BLOOD BANK CONTAINS many potentially dangerous materials, but the most hazardous substance to which employees are exposed may well be the blood itself. Despite careful screening and limited physical examinations, blood drawn from apparently healthy donors can contain infectious agents. Moreover, all blood components made from donor blood, including frozen products, are capable of transmitting infectious agents.

In addition to blood and its processed components, certain reagents used in laboratory testing may contain infectious material. The most obvious example of this are positive control sera for hepatitis B surface antigen testing. These products are obtained from human donors whose blood is positive for the hepatitis B surface antigen.

Other reagents used in the blood bank, which include reagent red blood cells as well as blood grouping sera, are derived from material found nonreactive for hepatitis B surface antigen (HBsAg) when tested with licensed reagents. However, as the label required by Food and Drug Administration (FDA) regulations asserts, no known test method can offer assurance that products derived from human blood will not transmit hepatitis.[1]

Having acknowledged the potential for reagents to transmit hepatitis, the potential for transmission of other agents, particularly human immunodeficiency virus (HIV), becomes a realistic concern. At present it is standard for American manufacturers to prepare reagents from blood that has tested negative for antibodies to HIV by an FDA-approved method.

Having ascertained that the blood bank is filled with material which can potentially transmit infectious disease, our next con-

Serl E. Rosenschein, MD, Pathologist, San Jose Hospital, San Jose, California

cern is to identify the employees who are at risk. All blood bank workers who handle either the patient, his or her blood or objects potentially contaminated with blood or serum, are at risk for acquiring an infectious disease. Consequently, nurses, physicians, laboratory technologists, technicians, phlebotomists, housekeepers, maintenance personnel and laundry workers are at risk. Clerical workers who handle paperwork soiled with blood or serum can also contact infectious agents, although the likelihood of significant infection is less.

Nurses or phlebotomists who perform venipuncture on donors or patients have the highest risk of needlestick injury. In the blood bank setting, such injuries are the most likely source of transmission of infectious agents. The transfer of infection by touching contaminated surfaces or handling contaminated objects does not often occur.

Specific Infectious Agents in the Blood Bank

Of the many infectious agents present in the blood bank, viruses are most numerous, and of the viral agents, those that transmit hepatitis are the most common. At least three different viruses cause hepatitis or inflammation of the liver: hepatitis A virus (HAV), hepatitis B virus (HBV) and an uncharacterized virus or group of viruses known as non-A,non-B hepatitis (NANB) virus.

Hepatitis A

Hepatitis A is caused by a 27-nanometer ribonucleic acid (RNA) virus. Transmission of this picornavirus occurs primarily by the fecal-oral route and is frequent when sanitation is poor and there is close contact between infected persons. Common source exposures from contamimated food and water also occur. The infection is rarely transmitted by blood products, although isolated cases have been reported.[2]

In short, transmission of hepatitis A infection in the blood bank setting is unusual and should be prevented by frequent hand washing.

Hepatitis B

Hepatitis B infection is caused by a 42-nanometer deoxyribonucleic acid (DNA) virus belonging to the class known as

Hepadna viruses. Despite the fact that the virus has not been grown in tissue culture, much is known about its structure and epidemiology.

Intact HBV is found in the serum of acutely and chronically infected persons. The surface of the 42-nanometer virus is composed of HBsAg, a 22-nanometer sphere or tubule. Large quantities of this surface protein are released into the serum during HBV infection. HBsAg usually appears from 1-2 months before the onset of symptoms, and 40-180 days after exposure.

Several subtypes of HBsAg exist, and these are of epidemiological interest. All HBsAg subtypes contain the *a* determinant and either the *d* or *y* and the *w* or *r* determinant. In the United States and Western Europe, *adw* is the most common subtype among chronic carriers, hence among blood donors.[3]

Hepatitis B envelope antigen (HBeAg) also appears in serum at the time that HBsAg is first detected. It persists for less time than HBsAg in the majority of patients. HBeAg is a reliable and sensitive serologic marker for the presence of high levels of virus, and therefore a high degree of infectivity. HBsAg-positive individuals who are HBeAg positive are highly infectious; they have a higher absolute number of infectious viral particles in their serum.

As HBeAg disappears from the serum, antibody to it (anti-HBe) develops. This seroconversion generally occurs at the peak of clinical symptoms and suggests that the disease is on the wane. Persons who progress to the chronic HBsAg carrier state do not seroconvert from HBeAg to anti-HBe during this phase of acute infection. The persistence of HBeAg by radioimmunoassay for more than 10 weeks is associated with the carrier state and with chronic-persistent or chronic-active hepatitis.[4]

In addition to HBsAg and HBeAg, there is HBcAg, or core antigen, the 27-nanometer nucleocapsid core found in the nuclei of liver cells infected with HBV. Under normal conditions, it is not found free in serum. However, anti-HBc is found in serum, appearing 2-4 weeks after HBsAg is first detected.

The final serologic marker of HBV infection is anti-HBs. It does not arise until the convalescent period. In all but a few patients, anti-HBs is not detectable in serum until HBsAg has disappeared and recovery is complete. Therefore, anti-HBs is a marker of recovery and immunity.

Hepatitis B infection is spread almost exclusively by the parenteral route or by intimate sexual contact. Serologic markers of prior hepatitis B infection are common among multiply transfused individuals, drug addicts, medical personnel and dialysis patients. Only about 50% of persons with acute type B hepatitis give a history of known parenteral exposure, even after close and thorough questioning. In these cases, inapparent parenteral spread probably occurred, such that the virus enters the body through a tiny insignificant break in the skin or mucous membrane. HBV does not seem capable of crossing the intact skin. Experimental studies have shown that the virus has extremely low infectivity by oral, nasal or respiratory routes.[5]

Health-care professionals who handle blood frequently are at an increased risk of contracting hepatitis B compared to the general population. Several surveys have confirmed this increased risk.[6] In one, 26% of blood bank workers demonstrated serologic markers indicative of previous HBV infection. In contrast, only 14% of dentists,[7] 10% of intensive care nurses,[6] and 4% of hospital workers with no patient contact have evidence of prior hepatitis B.[8] Five percent (5%) of all volunteer blood donors have previously been infected with HBV.[6]

Non-A,Non-B Hepatitis

Non-A,non-B (NANB) hepatitis is now known to be the most common form of posttransfusion hepatitis in the United States. It accounts for at least 80-90% of the reported cases.[9] Despite the fact that the disease was recognized a decade ago, the etiologic agent or agents have not been identified; consequently, no specific serologic test exists to identify persons infected with the virus. Recent reports have identified reverse transcriptase activity in sera of patients with non-A,non-B hepatitis, suggesting that the infectious agent may be a retrovirus.[10]

NANB hepatitis can apparently be transmitted by both systemic (ie, parenteral) and nonsystemic routes. Sporadic or community acquired cases are frequent and include spread within families or institutions. These cases, which are often mild or asymptomatic, probably account for the majority of carriers whose blood transmits the infection to transfusion recipients.

Certain surrogate or indirect tests exist for identifying potential carriers of NANB hepatitis. Recipients of blood that tests positive for anti-HBc have a two- to threefold greater risk of acquiring NANB hepatitis than recipients of blood without this marker.[11] Elevated ALT (alanine aminotransferase) levels in donors also correlate with an increased incidence of NANB hepatitis in their recipients.[12] Nevertheless, neither of these tests are specific and neither will detect all carriers of the virus. Moreover, a certain proportion of healthy donors who are not carriers of the virus will be excluded from the donor pool.

Since NANB hepatitis is the most frequent transfusion-associated disease, it stands to reason that the agent(s) causing the infection are the most frequently encountered viruses in the blood bank. We have shown that there is no specific test to identify blood from carriers of this virus, and therefore, it is only sensible to treat all blood specimens as if they contain NANB hepatitis—with extreme care.

Cytomegalovirus

Cytomegalovirus (CMV) belongs to the Herpes virus group. It is an enveloped, double-stranded DNA virus whose capsid displays icosahedral symmetry and consists of 162 capsomeres.[13] Like other Herpes viruses, CMV is capable of producing latent infection. Most evidence points to mononuclear cells, specifically lymphocytes, as the site of CMV latency.[14]

It is well-known that whole blood or leukocytes from asymptomatic individuals can transmit CMV infection.[14] Extensive efforts to isolate this virus from stored bank blood have not been successful, supporting the hypothesis that the virus is transmitted in a latent state, not actively replicating. CMV infection can cause immunosuppression and has been associated with "postperfusion syndrome." The syndrome was first described following coronary bypass procedures, but can occur after any blood transfusion. It seems to be particularly common following administration of large amounts of fresh blood. The syndrome manifests itself clinically 2-7 weeks after transfusion when the patient develops a mononucleosis-like disease. The symptoms and signs include fever, lymphadenopathy, hepatosplenomegaly, atypical lymphocytes in the peripheral blood and occasional skin rash.[15]

Epstein-Barr Virus

Epstein-Barr virus (EBV) belongs to the Herpes virus group. It is a 150- to 200-nanometer virus containing double-stranded DNA. It exists as an intracellular agent, commonly in the B lymphocytes of humans. EBV is the agent responsible for infectious mononucleosis and is closely linked to Burkitt's lymphoma and nasopharyngeal carcinoma. It has been known since 1969 that blood transfusions can transmit EBV infections.[16] Post-transfusion EBV can resemble hepatitis or the postperfusion syndrome. These transfusion-transmitted infections appear to be of significant risk only for immunodeficient patients.[17]

Human Immunodeficiency Virus

Human immunodeficiency virus (HIV), formerly known as human T-cell lymphotropic virus, type III (HTLV-III) or lymphadenopathy-associated virus (LAV), is a deadly retrovirus that captured the attention of the blood bank community in 1982. At that time, clinical and epidemiologic evidence mounted, linking the transmission of acquired immune deficiency syndrome (AIDS) to blood transfusion.[18] HIV is a retrovirus that was isolated in 1983 from patients with lymphadenopathy. It belongs to the same family as HTLV-I and II, which cause T-cell leukemia or lymphoma. The virus is an RNA virus that produces a magnesium-dependent reverse transcriptase. The HIV virus, like many others, is quite selective in the cell which it infects. Its cell of choice is the T-4 or T-helper cell, which is recognized as a pivotal cell for initiating the entire immune response. Infection with HIV can cause AIDS, AIDS-related complex (ARC) or subclinical infection. Most cases of HIV infection have been confined to so-called high risk groups, including homosexual or bisexual men, hemophiliacs or intravenous drug abusers. However, the infection has been described in women as well as infants and children. Infection can occur through parenteral exposure, by the transplacental route as well as through heterosexual intercourse. No cases of casual spread have been identified.

As our knowledge has increased regarding the transmission of the HIV agent, we have been able to confirm that the risk of nosocomial transmission is extremely low.[19]

The literature now contains a number of reports describing health-care workers who have had either direct parenteral or mucous membrane exposure to blood or other body fluids from AIDS patients and have not seroconverted.[20-23] The Centers for Disease Control (CDC) has followed over 938 cases of health-care personnel with such documented exposures. Follow-up periods averaged 15 months. Eighty-five percent of these exposures were to blood or serum, and 76% involved needlestick injuries or cuts with sharp implements. None of these 938 incidents resulted in the acquisition of signs or symptoms of the acquired immune deficiency syndrome.[19] The CDC has stated that the risk of transmission of hepatitis B virus infection to health-care workers is far greater than the risk of HIV transmission. Following a needlestick injury, the risk of acquiring HBV varies from 6-30%.[24] A similar injury results in a risk of HIV infection of less than 1%.[19]

Miscellaneous Viruses

Theoretically, almost any viral agent can be transmitted by blood. These viruses include the Delta agent (a defective virus that requires HBV to replicate), yellow fever virus, Marburg virus and other exotic tropical viruses. In reality, such infections are extraordinarily rare.

More anxiety has been expressed regarding the possibility of slow virus transmission by blood transfusion. Slow viruses include the agent that causes Creutzfeldt-Jakob disease. Documentation of transmission of this agent by biologic materials is present; however, there is no evidence that the disease has ever been transmitted by blood transfusion.

One cannot feel entirely complacent about this potential danger. Because these slow viruses remain latent for many years, it would take a long prospective study to truly evaluate the risk of transmission. There is a single study of 237 infants who received fetal or neonatal blood transfusions and were evaluated 3-7 years later. None of these children developed an illness that could be linked to a slow virus.[25,26]

Spirochetes

Treponema pallidum, the etiologic agent of syphilis, can theoretically be transmitted through fresh blood components. Today, posttransfusion syphilis is of only historical interest for two reasons. The first of these is the result of the use of stored, refrigerated bank blood rather than fresh blood. The second is the routine required testing of all donor blood with a serologic test for syphilis before it can be released from the blood bank.

Treponema pallidum is a spirochete measuring 5-20 microns in length. The agent is quickly destroyed by heating, drying, soap and water or changes in pH. Many studies have documented that *T. pallidum* cannot survive in stored human blood. As early as 1941, it was shown that human citrated blood stored at 4 C contained no viable spirochetes after 48 hours.[27]

Theoretically, syphilis could be transmitted by fresh blood from donors with active primary syphilis, since a serologic test for syphilis would be negative during the incubation period, despite the presence of spirochetes in the blood. Therefore, it is commonly believed that the use of refrigerated blood, rather than the routine use of a serologic test for syphilis, is responsible for the virtual absence of reported cases of posttransfusion syphilis. Theoretically at least, platelets that are stored for a short period of time and at room temperature are the component with the highest potential for transmitting syphilis.

Parasites

Of the parasitic infections transmitted by blood, malaria is the most common. Human malaria is caused by four species of *Plasmodium, P. falciparum, P. vivax, P. ovale* and *P. malariae.* In general, people are infected when the asexual sporozoites are injected into lymphatics or blood vessels during the bite of a carrier mosquito. Malaria usually results in a self-limited infection including fever, anemia, hypersplenism and edema. *P. falciparum* causes the most severe form of malaria, which not infrequently results in death.

The life cycle of all the species of *Plasmodium* parasites has two phases: a sexual cycle (sporogony) that takes place in the intestinal tract of the mosquito and an asexual cycle (schizogony) that occurs in the human host. When a person is bitten by an infected mosquito, the injected sporozoites enter the liver in a short period of time. There they begin to multiply in what is known as the exoerythrocyte cycle. Approximately 10 days later, small forms known as merozoites break out of the liver cells and are released into the circulation. There they seek out and penetrate the erythrocytes. Transfusion-associated malaria can only be acquired if intact red cells are present in the blood product. However, only a few parasites are necessary to transmit malaria. In 1949, Boyd documented the transmission of malaria with a dose of 10 parasites.[28] Transmission by accidental needlestick has been described in some instances.[29]

The incubation time for transfusion-transmitted malaria varies from approximately 8 days to 3 months (range of 1-110 days).[30] The viability of malaria organisms in blood, and hence their potential infectivity, declines after refrigerated storage for more than 7 days.

There is no practical serologic test to screen donors for malaria. The only effective tool to minimize bloodborne malaria transmission is accurate donor history. It is important for all physicians to be aware that transfusion does carry a potential risk of malaria transmission, however slight this may be. If this is common knowledge, the rare cases that are observed will not be misdiagnosed, and appropriate therapy will be quickly instituted.

Bacterial and Fungal Infections

Transmission of bacterial or fungal infections by blood transfusion occurs rarely in the United States because of several factors. First, blood is collected under sterile conditions into a closed system including sterile disposable plastic containers and tubing. Second, the universal storage of blood at refrigerated temperatures markedly decreases the count of viable bacteria even in units that have been contaminated. The likelihood of clinical infection following transfusion of viable organisms depends on the number of organisms transfused, the condition of the host and the pathogenicity of the organism.

After careful donor screening, it is unlikely that anyone suffering from bacteremia due to a pathogenic organism would be accepted as a blood donor. Therefore, the risk of contracting a significant bacterial, fungal or even rickettsial disease by accidental needlestick or splash exposure in the blood bank is extremely small.

Safety Precautions for Preventing Infection

It is prudent for all blood bank employees to pay careful attention to their personal safety while working with blood donors or their laboratory specimens. This includes constant awareness that any person, no matter how healthy he or she may appear, can harbor an infectious agent. The fear of acquiring AIDS has compelled health-care workers to be "extra careful" when caring for HIV-infected patients or their specimens. In fact, nurses and laboratory workers should be "extra careful" when caring for all patients and handling all clinical specimens, since it is impossible to determine with certainty which are infectious.

The safety measures recommended to prevent accidental transmission of hepatitis B, if followed, should prevent transmission of HIV or any other bloodborne pathogen. These precautions are summarized below and are in accordance with previously published guidelines.[31,32]

1. Specific coats, gowns or uniforms should be worn in the work place and changed weekly or after any overt contamination. Protective garments should not be worn in the lunchroom or outside the blood bank.
2. Any work garments that are contaminated by blood or other secretions should be carefully laundered, preferably in hot water and with household bleach.

3. All personnel performing activities that may involve skin contact with blood should be careful to protect any open cuts on their hands. Workers who have large areas of broken skin or dermatitis should wear gloves or should not perform activities that could result in blood contamination of the skin.

4. Hands should be washed frequently with soap and water. This practice should be routine after any direct contact with potentially infectious materials, even if gloves were worn.

5. Extreme care should be taken to avoid accidental wounds from needles or other sharp instruments.

6. Needles and other sharp instruments should be discarded into a puncture resistant container with a lid.

7. Needles should never be resheathed, purposefully bent, broken or otherwise manipulated by hand.

8. Any procedure that could result in the creation of droplets or aerosolization of blood should be performed with extreme care; if necessary, masks or goggles should be worn.

9. Whenever possible, specimens requiring centrifugation should first be placed into capped tubes. These should be placed into centrifuges that have a sealed dome. The centrifuge carriage should be treated daily with a germicide.

10. Mouth pipetting is forbidden. Mechanical pipetting devices should be used for the handling of *all* liquids in the laboratory.

11. All work surfaces should be decontaminated whenever spills occur and at the end of each day at the completion of work. Many chemical disinfectants are appropriate and are summarized in Table 4-1. Fresh solutions of sodium hypochlorite, which are made from one part household bleach containing 5.24% sodium hypochlorite and nine parts water, are especially effective and inexpensive.

12. All laboratory specimens and disposable items should be discarded in biohazard bags. When possible, these should be autoclaved prior to incineration or transportation to a hazardous waste facility.

13. If blood or serum accidentally contacts the skin, the area should be washed with an antimicrobial soap such as Hibiclens. After rinsing, a solution of household bleach in a 1:10 dilution or 50% isopropol or ethyl alcohol should be applied. After being allowed to remain on the skin for at least 1 minute, the area should again be washed with liquid soap and water.

Table 4-1. Chemical Agents Effective Against Human Immunodeficiency Virus*

Agent	Minimum Effective Concentration	Recommended Concentration†
Sodium hypochlorite	0.02%	0.5%
Sodium hydroxide	30 mM	30 mM
Glutaraldehyde	0.1%	1%
Formalin	2%	4%
Paraformaldehyde	0.5%	1%
B-propiolactone	1:400 dilution	1:400 dilution
Hydrogen peroxide	0.3%	1%
Ethyl alcohol	25%	50%
Isopropyl alcohol	30%	50%
Lysol	0.5%	1%
NP-40 detergent	1%	1%
Chlorhexidine gluconate/ ethanol mix	4/25%	4/25%
Quarternary ammonium chloride	0.08%	1%
Acetone/alcohol mix	1:1	1:1

*Used with permission from Tierno.[33]
†Recommended concentrations may be higher than minimum effective concentrations to ensure potency of these agents during clinical laboratory usage conditions.

Immunocompromised and Pregnant Employees

Whether direct patient or donor care should be given by an immunocompromised employee has become a concern for hospitals as well as blood centers, especially if the immunocompromised state is caused by HIV infection. In order to formulate an appropriate policy, one must consider the well-being of both the donor and the employee.

There is no epidemiological data indicating that transmission of AIDS from health-care worker to patient has ever occurred. Therefore, asymptomatic employees with HIV infection need not necessarily be restricted from work unless they have other infections or illnesses that might endanger others with whom they come in contact. An immunosuppressed employee could, theoretically at least, be at risk for acquiring an infection from a patient or specimen. For this reason, it is advisable to assign these employees to tasks where there is little likelihood of contact with microorganisms that could endanger their own health. Overall, each individual should be handled on a case-by-case basis.

It has been recommended that pregnant employees not engage in the direct care of AIDS patients who may shed cytomegalovirus in their body fluids.[34] CMV infection during pregnancy can cause birth defects, including mental retardation and deafness. The risk of transmission from infected patients to hospital personnel appears quite small as long as appropriate hygienic measures are followed. The risk of transmission in the blood bank setting should be even smaller. The CDC has formulated a general policy for those who participate in direct patient care. They maintain that patients infected with CMV can be identified and this information can then be used for counseling pregnant employees and determining their work assignments.[35]

Special Precautions for Housekeeping and Maintenance Workers

Housekeeping and maintenance workers should wear gloves when handling soiled laundry or other potentially infective material. If handling plastic bags that may contain broken glass or sharp instruments, heavy gloves are recommended.

Potentially infective waste should be contained and transported in clearly identified leakproof plastic bags. If the outside of the bag becomes contaminated with blood or other body fluids, a second outer bag should be used over the first. It is permissible to dispose of blood or body fluids by carefully pouring them down a drain that is connected directly to a sanitary sewer.

Housekeeping personnel are frequently responsible for cleaning, disinfection and sterilization procedures. Personnel who perform these procedures should be properly trained and wear appropriate protective garments.

Cleaning refers to the physical removal of organic material and microorganisms. Sterilization is defined as the destruction of all forms of microorganisms. Disinfection falls somewhere between the two and is mainly carried out through the use of chemical germicides.

Sterilization is recommended for nondisposable instruments that are introduced into the blood stream or other normally sterile parts of the body. When the nature of the material to be sterilized allows, steam sterilization is most effective as well as inexpensive.

Instruments that contact intact mucous membranes may be sterilized when possible. However, high level disinfection is adequate. A number of chemical germicides exist that can provide low, intermediate or high level disinfection. The level of disinfection achieved depends upon the nature of the contaminating organisms, contact time and temperature, as well as upon the type of germicide.

The United States Environmental Protection Agency (EPA) maintains a list of registered commercially available disinfectants. Those appropriate for high level disinfection are also known as "sterilants." In general, these are germicides that are mycobactericidal. They are preferred because mycobacteria are among the most resistant groups of microorganisms; therefore, any germicide effective against mycobacteria is probably effective against other bacterial and viral pathogens. In addition to other commercially available germicides, a freshly prepared solution of sodium hypochlorite, mentioned above, is very effective. Information on specific commercial germicides can be obtained from: Disinfectants Branch, Office of Pesticides, Environmental Protection Agency, 401 M Street SW, Washington, DC 20460.

Treatment of Employees Exposed to Infectious Agents

In the clinical and laboratory setting, an ounce of prevention is worth a pound of cure. The best way to handle accidental percutaneous or mucous membrane exposure to blood is to follow the safety guidelines established above and avoid the exposure. However, despite careful technique, accidents will occur.

After any needlestick injury or cut with a sharp instrument, the wound should be allowed to bleed freely. The injured area should be washed with soap and water. If the wound is small, a topical antiseptic or antibiotic cream may be applied. The area should then be covered by a dressing. This will prevent further contamination and protect against mechanical trauma, which could retard wound healing. An extensive injury may require sutures. In such cases, seek a physician's advice.

If the victim has never been immunized against tetanus or if the immunization history is unknown, tetanus vaccine should be administered, especially if the wound is deep.

Hepatitis B Exposure

Hepatitis B is the most significant laboratory-acquired infection for which effective preexposure and postexposure prophylactic measures exist. As noted previously, health-care workers with frequent blood contact are in a high risk group for acquiring hepatitis B infection. Therefore, the Public Health Service Immunization Practices Advisory Committee has recommended immunization with hepatitis B vaccine for susceptible individuals. Those who are already immune, who have anti-HBs and anti-HBc or only anti-HBs, do not require vaccination. All other employees with blood contact should receive the recommended three-dose regimen. This characteristically induces protective antibodies in over 90% of recipients. The recommended dose is 1.0 ml initially, followed by a second dose of 1.0 ml at 1 month and a third dose of 1.0 ml at 6 months.

The vaccine is manufactured from the pooled plasma of a-symptomatic individuals who are chronic hepatitis B carriers. There had been concern that the hepatitis B vaccine might transmit AIDS because some hepatitis B carriers are in high risk groups for AIDS. Studies have confirmed that HIV is not transmitted by the hepatitis B vaccine.[36]

Postexposure Prophylaxis

If a nonimmunized employee or one who has not completed the entire series of vaccinations sustains a percutaneous or mucous membrane exposure to blood that might contain HBsAg, a decision should be made about the administration of immune globulin. The decision depends upon the likelihood that the blood actually contains HBsAg and upon the type of exposure. In a hospital setting, the onset of clinical hepatitis B after exposure to blood containing HBsAg is approximately one in 20. The risk is about one in 2000 if the exposure is to blood of unknown HBsAg status. The recommendations for prophylaxis, therefore, are categorized based upon the following:
1. Whether the source of blood is known or unknown.
2. Whether the HBsAg status is known or unknown.[37]

Hepatitis B immune globulin (HBIG) should be given immediately if the known source of exposure is blood from an HBsAg-positive individual. The dose is 0.06 ml/kg, and this should be administered within 24 hours of exposure. After 1 month, a second identical dosage of globulin should be given.

If the source of the blood to which the employee was exposed is known, but the HBsAg status of the individual is unknown, a decision must be made as to whether or not the blood should be tested for HBsAg. In the blood bank setting, if the blood is from a donor, the testing is routine. If the result of the HBsAg test is negative, no prophylaxis for hepatitis B should be administered.

Whether or not administration of immune serum globulin (ISG) may provide protection against the development of NANB hepatitis is controversial. If a decision is made to administer immune globulin under these circumstances, ISG in a dose of 0.06 ml/kg should be given promptly. No further therapy is recommended.[37]

When an employee sustains an injury and the source of the blood is unknown, such as a cut from a broken test tube carelessly tossed in the garbage, it is virtually impossible to perform a test for the presence of HBsAg. In the blood bank setting, it is most likely that this blood came from a "healthy donor." Therefore, the likelihood of such blood being HBsAg positive is low. In such cases, prophylaxis is optional. If an immune globulin is administered, it should be immune serum globulin (ISG) at a dose of 0.06 ml/kg. This should be given as soon as possible, within 24 hours.

Storage and Shipment of Infectious Material

Storage of Infectious Material

Specimens from donors or patients, or any reagent that could contain an infectious material should be carefully stored in areas where spillage is unlikely to occur. These areas should be carefully labeled. Food or beverages must not be stored in the same refrigerator with specimens or reagents.

Shipping Protocols for Biohazardous Substances

On occasion, a blood bank may be required to transport hazardous materials by aircraft or other public transport. At least two separate sets of rules and regulations exist covering such shipment. The first is the *Code of Federal Regulations*, 49 CFR 100-177 and 42 CFR 72. The second set of regulations concerns air traffic and is published by the International Air Transport Association (IATA). Both FDA and IATA regulations apply to biological products as well as diagnostic specimens. Materials are exempt from special packaging rules only if they do not contain or are reasonably believed not to contain any infectious substances.

If transporting blood or serum that may contain viable microorganisms or their toxins, such as hepatitis B virus or HIV, special packaging standards apply.

Small Packages

If the total volume is less than 50 ml, the material should be placed in a securely closed, watertight primary container. This must then be enclosed in a second durable watertight container. More than one primary container (eg, vial or test tube) may be used as long as the total volume of all primary containers is less than 50 ml. The space at the top, bottom and sides between the primary and secondary containers should contain enough absorbant material to absorb the entire contents of the primary containers if leakage should occur.

The set of primary and secondary containers must be enclosed in an outer shipping carton constructed of corrugated fiberboard, cardboard, wood or other material of equivalent strength.

Large Packages

If the total volume is greater than 50 ml, some additional regulations apply. A shock absorbant material equal in volume to the volume of the absorbant material must be placed at the top, bottom and sides between the secondary container and the shipping container. No single primary container can hold more than 1000 ml of material. The outer shipping carton can contain no more than 4000 ml of material.

Specifications for outer shipping containers exist, but are too extensive to cover in this chapter. Potentially infectious material must be labeled as shown in Fig 4-1 or 4-2.

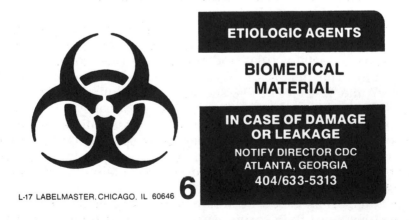

Figure 4-1. Biomedical material label required by federal regulations.

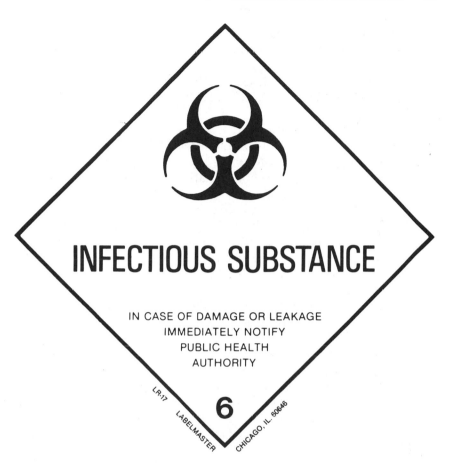

Figure 4-2. Infectious substance label required by IATA regulations.

References

1. Code of Federal Regulations, Title 21, part 606.120. Washington, DC: US Government Printing Office, 1985.
2. Meyers JD, Huff JC, Holmes KK et al. Parenterally transmitted hepatitis A associated with platelet transfusions. Ann Intern Med 1974;81:145-51.
3. Tabor E. Hepatitis as a complication of blood transfusion in infectious complications of blood transfusion. New York: Academic Press, 1982:7.
4. Aldershide J, Frosner GG, Nielsen JO et al. Hepatitis B antigen and antibody measured by RIA in acute hepatitis B surface antigen positive hepatitis. J Infect Dis 1980;141:293-8.

5. Hoofnagle JH. Types A and B viral hepatitis in perspectives on viral hepatitis. Chicago: Abbott Diagnostics Division, 1981:6.
6. Dienstag JL, Ryan DM. Occupational exposure to hepatitis B virus in hospital personnel: infection or immunization. Am J Epidemiol 1982;115:26.
7. Mosley JW, Edwards VM, Casey G et al. Hepatitis B virus infection in dentists. N Engl J Med 1975;293:729.
8. Denes, AE, Smith JL, Maynard JE et al. Hepatitis B infection in physicians. Results of a nationwide seroepidemiologic survey. JAMA 1978;239:210.
9. Gitnick G. Non-A, non-B hepatitis in perspectives on viral hepatitis. Chicago: Abbott Diagnostics Division, 1981:1.
10. Seto B, Coleman WG, Iwarson S et al. Detection of reverse transcriptase activity in association with non-A, non-B hepatitis agent(s). Lancet 1984;2:941-3.
11. Stevens CE, Aach RD, Hollinger B et al. Hepatitis B virus antibody in blood donors and the occurrence of non-A, non-B hepatitis in transfusion recipients. Ann Intern Med 1984;101:733-8.
12. Aach RD, Szmuness W, Mosley JW et al. Serum alanine amino-transferase of donors in relation to the risk of non-A, non-B hepatitis in recipients: the transfusion transmitted viruses study. N Engl J Med 1981;304:989-94.
13. Smith JD, DeHarven E. Herpes simplex virus and human cytomegalovirus replication in WI-38 cells. J Virol 1974;945-56.
14. Rook AH, Quinnan GV. Cytomegalovirus infections following blood transfusion. In: Tabor E, ed. Infectious complications of blood transfusion. New York: Academic Press, 1982:45-63.
15. Kreel I, Zoroff LI, Cantes JW et al. A syndrome following total body perfusion. Surg Gynecol Obstet 1960;111:317-21.
16. Gerber P, Walsh JH, Rosenblum EN et al. Association of EB-virus infection with the post-perfusion syndrome. Lancet 1969;1:593-6.
17. Henle W, Henle G. Epstein-Barr virus and blood transfusions. In: Dodd RY, Barker LS. Infection immunity and blood transfusion. New York: Alan R. Liss, Inc, 1985:201-9.
18. Centers for Disease Control. Possible transfusion associated acquired immune deficiency syndrome (AIDS). MMWR 1982;31:652-4.
19. McCray E. The cooperative needlestick surveillance group: special report. Occupational risk of the acquired immunodeficiency syndrome among health care workers. N Engl J Med 1986;314:1127-32.

20. Weiss SH, Saxinger WC, Richtman D et al. HTLV-III infection among health care workers: association with needle-stick injuries. JAMA 1985;254:2089-93.
21. Anonymous. Needlestick transmission of HTLV-III from a patient infected in Africa. Lancet 1984;2:1376-7.
22. Henderson DK, Saah AJ, Zak BJ. Risk of nosocomial infection with human T-cell lymphotropic virus type III/lymphadenopathy-associated virus in a large cohort of intensively exposed health care workers. Ann Intern Med 1986;104:644-7.
23. Stricof RL, Morse DL. HTLV-III/LAV seroconversion following a deep intramuscular needlestick injury. N Engl J Med 1986;314:1115.
24. Centers for Disease Control. Recommendations for preventing transmission of infection with HTLV-III/LAV in the workplace. MMWR 1985;34:681-3.
25. Turner JH, Hutchinson DL, Petriciani JC. Chimerism following fetal transfusion. Scand J Haematol 1973;10:358-66.
26. Turner JH, Hutchinson DL, Hayashi TT et al. Fetal and maternal risks associated with intrauterine transfusion procedures. Am J Obstet Gynecol 1975;123:251-6.
27. Tabor E. Transfusion-transmitted treponemal infection. Infectious complications of blood transfusion. New York: Academic Press, 1982:87-92.
28. Boyd MF. Malariology, Vol. 1. Philadelphia: WB Saunders, 1949.
29. Bruce-Chwatt LJ. Essential malariology. New York: John Wiley and Sons, Inc, 1985.
30. Kark JA. Malaria transmitted by blood transfusion. In: Tabor E. Infectious complications of blood transfusion. New York: Academic Press, 1982:93-126.
31. Centers for Disease Control. Acquired immune deficiency syndrome (AIDS): precautions for clinical and laboratory staffs. MMWR 1982;31:577-80.
32. Centers for Disease Control. Acquired immunodeficiency syndrome (AIDS): precautions for health care workers and allied professionals. MMWR 1983;32:450-1.
33. Tierno M. Preventing acquisition of human immunodeficiency virus in the laboratory: safe handling of AIDS specimens. Lab Med 1986;17:696-8.
34. Safai B. Safety precautions for dealing with AIDS. In: DeVita VT, Helman S, Rosenberg SA, eds. AIDS: etiology, diagnosis, treatment and prevention. Philadelphia: JB Lippincott, 1985:269.
35. Williams WW. CDC guideline for infection control in hospital personnel. Infect Control 1983;4:326-49.

36. Centers for Disease Control. Hepatitis B vaccine: evidence confirming lack of AIDS transmission. MMWR 1984; 33:685-7.
37. California State Department of Health Services. Control of communicable diseases in California. 1983:228.

Suggested Reading

1. Infection control in the hospital. 4th ed. Chicago: American Hospital Association, 1979.
2. Centers for Disease Control. Inactivated hepatitis B virus vaccine. Ann Intern Med 1982;97:379-83.

Index